THE ART OF LEARNED RELAXATION

YOGA FOR DEPRESSION AND ANXIETY

GORDON KANZER, MD

Dedicated to the memory of my sweet Bella

Her unconditional love helped me through the most difficult of times

CONTENTS

Introduction   vii

PART I
THE ART OF LEARNED RELAXATION

1. Yoga Stills the Fluctuations of the Mind: An
   Overview   3
2. Depression and Anxiety: It's What You Have,
   Not Who You Are!   23
3. What is Relaxation and How to Achieve It   41
4. The Body-Mind Connection and Relaxation   65
5. A Healthier Body   81
6. A Healthier Mind   95
7. The External World and the Internal Self   123
8. The Love of Wisdom and the Love of Self   145

PART II
THE PRACTICE OF LEARNED RELAXATION

9. Stretching Into Relaxation   179
10. Posture Sequences to De-Stress   219
11. A Time to Let Go   297
12. Breathing Into Relaxation   305
13. Calming the Storm   337
14. The Coda   347

Afterword   355
Appendix   357
About the Author   363
Also by Gordon Kanzer, MD   365

INTRODUCTION

My primary intention as a physician, yoga instructor and author has always been to help people find themselves in a better place. I do not know you personally, but my own mental challenges allow me to have empathy for any pain you might be experiencing. Quite simply, I care for you and, therefore, it is absolutely necessary to begin this book with what I feel are the most important words that I will write:

> *If at this time, you find yourself in a dark place, please reach out to loved ones, friends, professionals or others for support. I have been in that dark place and I can assure you that eventually the psychic pain resolves and feelings of desperation abate. A suicide attempt is often a cry for help. Before you get to that point, make sure you cry out loudly to all of those that can offer their help, support and love. They are depending on it!*

<u>Dialing 988</u> is a direct link to:

The National Suicide Prevention Hotline

https://suicidepreventionlifeline.org.

You will be able to talk to a caring, nonjudgmental person.

Awareness of the breath is a large part of learned relaxation. So, now take a deep breath and then please read the above words one more time. Even if they don't apply to you, you will be able to pass them along to those who are in need. They will be grateful that you did.

There are general commonalities in the experiences of those that suffer from depression and anxiety. Each reader of this book, however, has different perspectives, life experiences, emotional sensitivities to concepts and words, varying physical abilities and limitations, and differing emotional states. I sincerely wish for you to find some peace, solace and an improved sense of wellbeing through the practice of yoga. In any attempt to do so, however, connecting with yourself is paramount to prevent any harm to either body or mind.

With regard to the body, if a particular movement or position causes discomfort or pain, modify your practice. You must listen to your body. Enter into your yoga practice with a full understanding of your physical limitations and any predispositions to injury you may possess. Contraindications are medical conditions that disqualify someone from doing an activity. In the back of this book, I have included an appendix of some of the more common contraindications to the performance of the *asanas*, or poses, and *pranayama,* or the breathing techniques. Before considering any postures or breathing techniques that are unfamiliar to you, I strongly recommend that you consult the appendix. Since this is not meant to be an exhaustive, fully comprehensive list, if you do have any questions or concerns about any physical or medical issues that are not included in the appendix or unsure about the potential physical detriment of any condition, I highly recommend that you consult with a physician or other medical professional.

With regard to the mind, it is an unrealistic expectation that every posture or breathing technique will improve your mental state. If there are certain *asanas* or *pranayama* that make you feel uncomfortable or you simply dislike, do not feel compelled to do them. Yoga offers many different paths toward wellbeing. Your path doesn't necessarily need to pass though anything that doesn't suit you. In addition, I'm just a guide making suggestions. You are experiencing my version of yoga and my thoughts, neither of which may speak to you. If any of my words trigger disturbing thoughts, are emotionally uncomfortable or elicit images of past traumas, please do not read any further or skip to some other paragraph or chapter.

I do not know you, but your interest in this book tells me that we both face some sort of mental challenge. I ultimately cannot be responsible for your experience, but I deeply care about your experience. In the hope that my words will resonate with you, I must accept the responsibility to be true to my authentic self and open about my mental illness in my attempt to describe yoga as one path toward mental wellness.

Realistic expectations are necessary when reading this book. Most importantly, yoga is not a cure for mental illness. Rather, it is an effective coping mechanism that complements other therapies that also promote mental wellness. It is a wonderful relaxation technique with the potential for personal growth, a spiritual connection and self-discovery. Yoga should be embraced to help you cope with whatever mental challenges you may face, but without abandoning other therapies that you may be receiving.

In addition, since I have no certified training in psychiatry, psychology or psychotherapy, my words must be read in the context of a radiologist, a yoga instructor, and someone with firsthand knowledge of mental disease. As a radiologist, I possess a comprehensive knowledge of human anatomy, a deep understanding of the physiological changes that occur with learned relaxation and an appreciation for the emerging science regarding the health benefits of yoga. As a certified yoga instructor trained in the Kripalu tradition, a yogic philosophy based in self-kindness, I possess knowledge of the *asanas* and *pranayama* and the many sides of yoga, including its philosophy and tenets. Through my own practice, I have also realized the many benefits of yoga, including stress reduction, increased physical strength and flexibility, and greater peace of mind. As a person who has suffered a lifetime with depression and anxiety and has received numerous treatments with limited success, I know of the challenges and frustrations inherent to mental disease. I also know how it feels when the mind clears of negative thoughts and rumination to allow me to better appreciate the blessings in my life. I hope to provide you with a direct approach to cope better with whatever mental challenges you face by melding the principles and ideas from these three worlds I know so well: medicine, yoga and mental disease. Most importantly, my experiences allow me to write from the heart with extreme empathy and a deep concern for you, the reader.

This book consists of two parts. The first part approaches learned relaxation from a variety of perspectives to establish a base of knowledge on which you may build, along with strategies for effectively coping with depression and anxiety. The second part presents the practical applications of yoga that foster states of relaxation in the context of your newfound knowledge and understanding.

Most importantly, please read my words as those of someone who cares. I have always cherished anyone and anything that supported and helped me cope with my own pain. My hope is that this book will instill within you a love for yoga and, with that love, allow you to cherish the blessings that life has to offer.

I write with gratitude. I am grateful for you entrusting me to be your guide into the world of yoga and humbled by your desire to read my words. Yoga is a gift I gave myself. Now, I wish to give it to you!

PART I

THE ART OF LEARNED RELAXATION

1

YOGA STILLS THE FLUCTUATIONS OF THE MIND: AN OVERVIEW

Yogash chitta vritti nirodhah is an aphorism written by Pantanjali in *The Yoga Sutras,* a seminal book that laid the foundation for all classical yogic philosophy to follow. Translated from the Sanskrit, it means, "yoga stills the fluctuations of the mind." Although written centuries ago, it continues to embody the true essence of yoga: the attainment of clarity of mind and spirit.

Imagine your mind a pond. Depression and anxiety are like stones that you toss that create ripples along the surface of the water. For some, those stones are small pebbles and, for some, large rocks. Those ripples are quite visible, but need not define you. The practice of yoga has the power to smooth out the ripples. And as they disappear, the unique and special person you are becomes visible below the surface. Yoga allows us to see deep down into the soul, connecting to thoughts, ideas and emotions.

Yogash chitta vritti nirodhah can become a powerful mantra in the battle against depression and anxiety. In order to access states of relaxation, one must learn how to still an active mind. Yoga provides the tools to master learned relaxation. Learned relaxation might be considered a "skill" that can be used to lessen the impact of these often debilitating diseases. Rather, I believe an "art" is a better qualifier since the learning process requires creativity, the imagination, and self-reflection. Similar to a successful artist, you can create your own version of yoga that comes from the heart, based on life experiences and imbued with individuality and uniqueness. Once this art is mastered, states of relaxation can be accessed at any time, especially when the symptoms of anxiety and depression are at their worst. You will learn to have some control over what you thought you never could.

Of course, this is all easier said than done. It requires work and patience and, most importantly, a dedication to self-kindness. The hope is that repeated reinforcement of self-kindness in your yoga practice will carry over to enhance your life experiences. Often inherent to depression and anxiety is an apparent need to beat oneself up for perceived weaknesses and shortcomings. Quite simply, the acceptance of self in your yoga practice without judgment opens up a new opportunity to become a good friend to yourself.

The subject of this book is complex, but its premise is

simple: learning to appreciate what exists in the present in order to access states of relaxation. More specifically, relaxation is realized by generating, sustaining and focusing on a single thought or idea that relates to whatever you are doing in the moment. Ruminating on regrets of the past, worries about the future and the pain and suffering inherent to depression and anxiety creates mental static, noise that clouds the mind and disrupts concentration. Disturbing thoughts elicit stress and anxiety, which often fuel a negative feedback loop of more disturbing thoughts with more stress and anxiety. Learned relaxation is the brake that slows an active, unproductive mind, allowing it to experience and witness the moments that have been quickly passing you by. You see where you are, not where you were or where you are going.

The process of learned relaxation is training the brain to focus on an idea or string of thoughts that pertain to what is occurring in the present. It is facilitated by tapping into all yoga has to offer. A mindfulness-based yoga practice requires using all of the senses to gain awareness of the experience of the physical body at any given moment. Although on the face of it, it seems that we are focusing on a particular physical sensation, such as the contact points of the body on the mat using the sense of touch, in actuality we are focusing on the thought that is created by the brain's interpretation of that physical sensation. As such, we can focus on any thought that is concerned with what we are doing at any given moment. Those thoughts might include novel ideas that come from the principles of yogic philosophy, human physiology and science or your own emotions and thoughts that pertain to a particular pose or breathing technique in which you are engaged. Whatever thought your choice of single-pointed focus might be, it is appreciated in the context of a particular *asana*, or pose, that you are assuming in the present moment. Heightened awareness of the breath is also a powerful way to achieve undistracted concentration. Listening to the sound of the breath moving in and out of the nose or connecting the breath to one's unique movements can induce meditative states. Regardless of the source of ideas or thoughts, their relation to the present diverts one's attention away from more disturbing, stressful issues that press down upon the spirit. Freeing the spirit to explore new possibilities is at the heart of learned relaxation.

As you assume a particular *asana* in your yoga practice, innumerable points of focus become apparent like an expansive, moonless night sky full of stars. As yoga is a personal experience, the choice of your focus of awareness is yours. To illustrate this, let us consider the *asana, virabhadrasana II*, or warrior II. You can approach the pose from many different perspectives to discover that which best promotes single-pointed concentration. You might become mindful of the sense of touch in gaining awareness of the points of contact of the feet on the mat. For warrior II, gaze is directed over the front hand. As such, using the sense of sight you can observe the qualities and features of the fingers or what might lie beyond in the distance. In addition, introducing novelty lessens the potential for mind chatter that often increases with familiarity. Bending a single finger of the visualized front hand directs all thought to that action. In fact, it is extremely difficult to focus on anything else other than that simple movement.

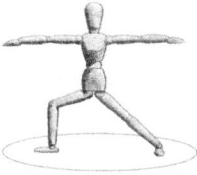

While in the warrior pose, you might also consider the philosophical principle of *santosha*. *Santosha* is Sanskrit for "contentment", which can be realized through self-acceptance of limitations. The strength of your warrior comes from pride in your abilities, not from lamentations on your inabilities. You could also choose to reflect on the ancient origins of yoga and the guiding principles of its philosophy found in the Hindu myth of the eponymous Virabhadra, a warrior created by the deity Shiva to avenge the death of his wife Sati. It is a story of remorse and the consequences of acting out rashly and impulsively.

Virabhadrasana II ~ Warrior II

Another unique perspective comes from a consideration of the physiology of the body while in *virabharasana*. Grounding is a guiding principle for all of the standing postures. Actively and evenly grounding the feet into the mat in the warrior results in contraction of the muscles of the legs. Muscular contraction requires a greater delivery of oxygen. Without sufficient oxygen, excess lactic acid accumulates in the muscles, which results in the "burn". We can all relate to this sensation in the thigh muscles as we climb a long flight of stairs. We increase the supply of oxygen through deep diaphragmatic breathing, which also activates the parasympathetic or "rest and digest" nervous system to promote relaxation. Knowledge of human physiology gives new meaning to the act of breathing.

The breath also has spiritual meaning, as it is a vehicle for receiving *prana*, the life force that surrounds us all. One can also choose to focus on the sound or sensation of air moving in and out of the nostrils or connecting inhalations and exhalations to one's unique movements.

Finally, the warrior pose can possess deep, personal meaning. Feelings of pride and strength, the qualities of a warrior, can arise from reflecting on any attempt to overcome challenges you face, or possibly challenges you have overcome. Since you are the one assuming a pose, exploration of a particular *asana* is actually a process of self-analysis; being the witness to your thoughts and emotions.

The aforementioned example illustrates just a few of the many aspects and meanings of an *asana* on which to focus to elicit novel, interesting ideas. A single pose can be approached from different perspectives, with a commonality that lies in their ability to stimulate the mind and create profound thought. That ability is heightened by changing your point of focus each time you assume a pose in the interest of keeping your yoga practice fresh, promoting self-inquiry.

As yoga is a practice, learning the ability to achieve single-pointed concentration takes time and patience. None of us possess a mental switch to turn off mind chatter. Once this ability is learned, however, clarity of mind ensues. Once clarity of mind is established, connecting to one's true authentic self and the ability to relax can be realized. And, the key to access everything that yoga has to offer is using your imagination, creativity and knowledge. You become your own teacher as you learn to relax. Relaxation quiets the storm of stress, anxiety and rumination as yoga becomes your sanctuary, within which are the tools to cope with depression and anxiety.

My hope is that by reading this book, you will achieve learned relaxation based in the present moment, whether it be through the practice of mindfulness of physical sensations, the application of knowledge or the connection of the breath to your unique movements. It is a process of substituting healthy actions, ideas and emotions for that which don't serve in the present. Through learned relaxation you will not only be in the moment, but you will possess a newfound power to cherish every moment. In the words of the Dalai Lama, "There are only two days in the year that nothing can be done. One is called yesterday and the other is called tomorrow. Today is the right day to love, believe, do and mostly live."

Stilling the fluctuations of the mind results in mental clarity, which is necessary for effective self-analysis. Rather than reacting emotionally to disturbing thoughts, one can become an objective witness in order to determine why regrets and worries possess so much power. For many, those emotional reactions are ingrained, reflexive defense mechanisms that have developed over many years. Automatic negative thoughts often manifest as cognitive distortions. Misinterpretations of reality deprive the mind of accurate information needed to react appropriately to daily interactions and experiences. This book will also delve into the content of these cognitive distortions, which once recognized can be disarmed of their emotional power. The mind has newfound freedom to substitute positive affirmations once true reality becomes apparent. Similar to the practice of yoga, learning to recognize automatic negative thoughts and substituting positive affirmations requires much patience. Setbacks will occur. We lack the ability to simply and quickly eliminate negative thoughts and enjoy positive ones. Developing mental flexibility from a rigid mind occurs very gradually over time.

Further, the expectation that learned relaxation though yoga will lead to a life filled with happiness and bliss will set you up to fail. The road of life is inherently a bumpy one with its ups and downs and successes and failures. Newfound mental clarity and self-analysis, however, will lead to a healthier emotional mind that will lessen the impact of those bumps in the road.

Self-analysis and the discovery of your true authentic self can be exciting, but at the same time stressful, as it takes courage to dismiss the expectations of others, how they wish you to be, and face true desires and emotions that may have been suppressed or repressed for years. Inserting periods of rest and stillness into a yoga practice enables the development of this intimate connection to self. It has been said, "The magic of yoga occurs in the spaces between the postures." That magic reveals the special person that you are, one that is not defined by mental illness. Depression and/or anxiety are what you have, not who you are.

Yoga is a journey. We need not be concerned, however, with our destination. Non-attachment to final outcomes is necessary to simply enjoy the process. Without expectations, you will progress further on your path with a healthy awareness of each step you take. For those that face mental challenges, following that path requires energy. Depression and anxiety deplete energy, causing mental paralysis in their most extreme forms. My hope is that this book will offer an array of different concepts that promote an active mind filled with newfound positive energy, which in turn will leave you better equipped to take action to battle the challenges you face.

One should have realistic expectations before embarking on the path to learned relaxation. Learning to live in the present by focusing on sensations through mindfulness, applying your newfound knowledge of yoga, and achieving states of introversion that promote self-analysis is the work to be done, but don't expect to be a master of it all. I have accepted that I will always be a work in progress. My depression and anxiety will likely never fully resolve. My expectation, however, is that my dedication to a meaningful yoga practice will lessen the impact of both diseases.

Learned relaxation will help you to better cope by smoothing out the ripples caused by depression and anxiety just enough to see what life has to offer. The cloud of depression and anxiety will clear and what will glisten in the sunshine beneath the surface will be all the blessings of your life. An appreciation for those blessings begins with gratitude. Gratitude is a prerequisite for all of the other positive emotions that we experience. From gratitude, feelings of pride, hope and joy become possible. It has been said, "Happiness does not bring gratitude, rather it is gratitude that brings happiness."

Most importantly, approach the work to be done with self-kindness. There is no need to chastise oneself for perceived failures. Be proud of yourself for your desire to read this book in the interest of self-care. Always try to be a friend to yourself. If a friend scrutinized or criticized everything you did, you would likely end that relationship. Be the good friend that unconditionally supports and loves you. Allow yoga to be the path to that love. Self-deprecation can be a defense mechanism that has been ingrained for years, with self-fulfilling prophecies of failure at its worst. Don't let those setbacks trigger generalized feelings of inadequacy. Always focus on what you can do and not what you can't.

With learned relaxation, you are teaching yourself the tools that will help you cope with the stress that fuels depression and anxiety. Don't be that mean teacher that ridicules students. Be the teacher that cherishes knowledge and opportunity. Try not to attach to a final outcome. Don't emphasize success or failure, which exist in the future. Rather, enjoy the process that exists in the present. In fact, removing the pressure to succeed or perform often increases the odds of success.

Eventually, through insight and reflection, a revelation may occur: you can have some control over what you thought you never could. That control occurs through deliberate relaxation. With patience, you can realize your place of peace, within which lies the ability to relax on conscious, subconscious, and spiritual levels.

I feel it is so very important to stress that yoga done on a regular basis can better facilitate the process of learned relaxation than if done sporadically. In that regard, developing the proper mindset is necessary to realize a regular, meaningful practice. When something "sets" it becomes rigid, hardened and fixed. A mindset is an attachment to one's fixed beliefs and habitual thoughts and behaviors. Changing one's mindset is a challenge, especially when it is mired in automatic and reflexive negative self-judgments. Developing the proper mindset and intentions is requisite before expectations for positive change through yoga can be considered. Practicing non-attachment to future outcomes and becoming mindful in the moment is part of the work that needs to be done to become more receptive to new ideas and perspectives. Perhaps, that receptivity allows the mind to remain fluid, preventing it from becoming rigid, hardened and fixed, not allowing the mind to "set". Embracing new perspectives can be both empowering and liberating.

A mindset driven by a need to perform, a fear of making mistakes, or perceived inadequacies will be an impediment to personal growth through a meaningful yoga practice. Returning to "the mind as a pond" metaphor, we can create additional ripples by tossing in negative self-judgments about limitations. The inner critic produces those ripples that prevent the appreciation of our positive qualities and life blessings that lie beneath the surface. Once again, yoga smooths the surface, returning peace and serenity to the pond.

The practice of self-kindness is called *ahimsa*. I will discuss this philosophical concept in greater detail in a later chapter. Suffice it to say, *ahimsa* refers to doing no harm by honoring body and mind. The former is accomplished by modifying one's practice to prevent injury and easing off from the edge where discomfort is experienced. The latter is accomplished through self-kindness and compassion.

In his writings, Thich Nhat Hanh tells of the Buddhist parable of the second arrow in the context of pain and suffering. Being hit by an arrow causes pain. If a second arrow enters in the same exact spot as the first, the pain is a significant magnitude greater. Awareness of limitations, either mental or physical, is the first arrow. Negative self-judgments and lamentations regarding those limitations are the second, clouding the mind with the power for them to become all-consuming.

In the practice of yoga, however, does there need to be a

first arrow? Does an awareness of limitations necessarily need to be emotionally painful or necessary at all? Even more so, are there actually any limitations to the practice of yoga? Of course, this is a rhetorical question. The *asanas* were created by someone at some point in time as a reliable way to communicate movements and postures from teachers to students and from one practitioner to another. Many of the poses we do today were created in the relatively recent past. Many of them began as Scandinavian gymnastic poses that were adopted by the British and subsequently brought to India during British colonization. As an expression of Indian nationalism, Sanskrit names and meanings and symbolism based in Hinduism were assigned to the *asanas*. In a sense, the creation of the *asanas* that we practice today was somewhat arbitrary. Therefore, I could make the argument that any position of my body that I choose to assume would classify as a yoga pose. So, how important is it to be able to do all of these established *asanas* perfectly, or even be able to do them at all? More important is to integrate the breath with your own unique movements to achieve meditative states. Part of learning to relax is developing this connection of the breath to movement. Clouding the mind with negative thoughts stemming from perceived limitations is quite simply not relaxing. When I tell people I am a yoga instructor, for many different reasons I commonly hear, "I can't do yoga". What does it mean to "do" yoga? If doing yoga is simply connecting the breath to movements, then the complete novice can have a more meaningful practice than the most advanced practitioner that doesn't find that connection. I often tell the story of a legally blind, handicapped woman in a chair yoga class I taught. She used a walker and was accompanied by an aide. She was unable to come out of her chair when I led the class through the standing postures, but followed along using her upper body movements. The question is, "if she was connecting her breath to those movements, was she doing yoga?" The answer is a categorical yes!

Our bodies all move in their own individual ways, relating to differences in inherited and acquired characteristics. As a yoga instructor, I might guide you into a particular *asana*. You may not be able to assume the pose as I can, but I assure you I will never be able to position my body exactly as you do. Thankfully, we are all unique. Yoga is not a game of Simon Says, but an exploration of one's own personal expression that takes the form of your movements connected to your breath.

It is critical to approach yoga with self-compassion. The enemy that can block any attempt at self-kindness, however, is the inner critic. It is the part of one's thinking that creates a cacophony of mind chatter filled with rumination over one's faults and shortcomings. Worsening the effects of the inner-critic are self-blame and perceived weakness that are inherent to depression and anxiety. Our inner critic stymies our efforts, minimizes our achievements, compares us to others, beats us up and bruises our self-esteem. The inner critic develops at a very early age when one has yet to develop the ability of abstract thought and the differentiation of right from wrong. We do not yet know that our parents are fallible, wrong at times and capable of mistakes. We accept everything they do or say as "right." Anything that sparks the expression of disapproval elicits feelings of shame and inadequacy in the young child. At a very young age, it is simply impossible to live up to what we perceive as our parents' ideals. Throughout childhood we will inevitably be confronted with parental disapproval. For some, that happens more often than for others, and perhaps for them, their inner critic represents a much more dominant and negative force later in their lives.

Feelings of low self-esteem and global negativity that can be symptoms of clinical depression are significantly worsened in the hands of the inner critic. Although easier said than done, learned relaxation through yoga requires silencing the inner critic as much as possible. One problem that can arise, however, is that your inner critic can be fueled by your inability to silence your inner critic. This is a so-called "catch-22". As you try to suppress undesirable, negative self-judgments, you begin to hate yourself for lacking the capacity to do so. In fact, the more you find you can't suppress the mind chatter, the louder the inner critic becomes, possibly so loud as to consume you. The solution is to realize it takes two to wage a war. Stop fighting with yourself. Congratulate yourself for taking the first step toward acceptance: awareness. Awareness results in the newfound ability to acknowledge the inner criticisms. When a self-critical thought arises, acknowledge it and then let it go as if you are throwing it into a river, watching it disappear downstream. In fact, you can even go so far as to embrace your inner critic. Love your enemy. The inner critic will attempt to make you feel "bad" for perceived inabilities and convince you that they disqualify you from being "good" at yoga. Don't believe everything it tells you. The inner critic can be proved wrong by eliminating preconceived notions of what it is to "do" yoga. Accept yourself for who you are. Will your inner critic ever leave? Probably not, but without the expenditure of all of the negative energy it takes to wage the war, the inner critic will become more and more quiet with time. With the acceptance that you are enough comes empowerment. You become empowered to make positive choices, choices that ultimately will allow you to embrace all the blessings in your life.

When I first began a regular yoga practice, two people showed up on my mat: me and my inner critic. Many of my negative self-judgments arose from my physical inflexibility that developed over thirty years of working in a stressful career. The misconception that yoga requires physical flexibility is an obstacle for those that aren't. Inflexibility can be acquired or inherited. We are all born with a certain range of motion in all of our joints that differs from person to person. The shape of men and women's pelvises differ. It may be that flexibility will be limited by the innate, restrictive, anatomical relationships in the body, preventing one from assuming certain positions, even after years of yogic practice. Due to inherited inflexibilities, I doubt that my knees will ever touch the ground in *supta baddha konasana* or reclining bound angle pose, which consists of lying supine with the soles of feet touching. As one lets their knees drop out laterally toward the floor, the groin spreads open and the hip adductor or inner thigh muscles are stretched. Can I still enjoy the stretch in my adductor muscles that this posture affords me even though my knees are up in the air? Absolutely! Should I lament my physical limitation as an obstacle to developing a meaningful yoga practice? Absolutely not! My self-observation without judgment consists of eliminating the word "and". Instead of, "My knees will never touch the ground and I will never be fully able to do this posture", I choose to alternatively say to myself, "My knees don't touch the ground." Or if I choose to use the word "and", "My knees don't touch the ground and I am enjoying breathing into the stretch in my inner thigh muscles". I accept that I don't possess the range of motion in my hip joints for my knees to drop all the way down to the mat. It is who I am. I inherited this particular trait just as I have dark brown hair. Fortunately, the word "modification" exists. Any yoga pose can be modified to suit the particular individual's physical situation. A modification is changing the expression of an *asana* to decrease discomfort or muscle strain. Modifying a pose can clear thoughts of discomfort that can cloud the mind. In the reclining bound angle pose, I might consider placing bolsters to support my knees so they need not dangle in the air. Of course, some of my hip adductor inflexibility has been acquired over many years of sitting in a chair throughout my career. I am overjoyed to say, however, that I have made a little progress in increasing my range of motion. Possibly, over time I will realize more flexibility, but I must be patient and realistic at the same time. Awareness and acceptance are key.

Arguably, more important than increasing range of motion in the physical body is the development of flexibility of the mind. We are so often set in our ways with fixed beliefs that have solidified over many years. Yoga affords time for self-reflection and analysis of one's belief system. Personal growth comes from becoming receptive to new ideas and possibilities and welcoming different perspectives.

As you practice yoga, always remember that you have choice. You can choose how to move, how to breathe, and how to treat yourself. I know from personal experience that being told to love yourself doesn't help much. It must come from within. I can't promise you that yoga will instill feelings of self-love and self-worth. I can say, however, that it is worth the attempt to see if those feelings are possible. I can be very honest. There are times that I don't like myself. But, there are also times that I am filled with gratitude and hope, emotions that I have learned to more easily access through yoga. Yoga has given me a wonderful opportunity for discovery and self-realization that has smoothed out the ripples and allowed me to see deep below the surface the person I want to be; a person of worth, deserved of love.

I often hear and read that in the practice of yoga we need to accept our limitations. The only true limitation is the failure to recognize the beauty of one's body as it uniquely flows through space and the inner beauty of one's spirit that lies deep down in the soul.

It is now time to move onward to a consideration of learned relaxation. Our journey begins with a consideration of what is meant by depression and anxiety, followed by a detailed examination of the mind and body and the connection of the two, the practice of mindfulness and the application of yogic philosophy to promote self-love and kindness. Once we have created this firm base of knowledge, we can then build our yoga practice upon it, as we embrace the experience of learned relaxation. As you read on, remember that I am just the author and that ultimately it is you, the reader, that possesses the power to create and direct your own journey that will best help you to cope with whatever challenges you face.

2

DEPRESSION AND ANXIETY: IT'S WHAT YOU HAVE, NOT WHO YOU ARE!

This is not a book about mental illness, but one about achieving mental wellness. Everyone's definition and experience of depression or anxiety is different, as it should be. For many of you, I need not explain what depression and anxiety feel like. You already know. Nonetheless, for those that might profit from more insight into these conditions, including significant others of those that do suffer, I thought it might be worthwhile to define depression and anxiety both in situational and clinical contexts before exploring the art of learned relaxation. Awareness and understanding of the complexities of a problem must precede the implementation of a solution.

To be certain, anxiety and depression are often vague terms. Our language is fraught with words that fall short in eliciting a full appreciation of a particular concept. We each tend to possess our own idea of the meaning of words based on our own life experiences.

With regard to depression, the Ancient Greeks called it melancholia, literally meaning "black bile", specifically an imbalance in the body's humors and a deep disturbance in the physiology of the mind and body. For some, depression includes feelings of despondency and dispiritedness. The intensity of these emotions and their impact on wellbeing differ from individual to individual regardless of whether they are situational, secondary to habitual cognitive distortions or manifestations of clinical depression. This segregation of etiologies, however, is artificial, as the cause of depression is multi-factorial. And, the magnitude of suffering is unrelated to its etiology. We also all possess different tolerances for pain and varying degrees of resiliency.

As I have mentioned, I have no formal training in psychiatry, psychology or psychotherapy. I thought, however, based on personal experience, my own review of research and my discussions with trained, board certified professionals and others who suffer, I might attempt to describe how it feels to suffer from clinical depression. I do not, nor does anyone else that is unfortunate enough to possess a diagnosis of depression, necessarily experience everything I will describe, but my hope is that it might provide an overall picture of a disease that is often beyond description.

Firstly, depression is not just feeling sad. Others' exhortations to simply "cheer up" or "you should think about all of the good things in your life" are ineffective and possess a lack of understanding of the complexities and magnitude of the disease. Rather, depression is a state of unrelenting psychic pain that seems to arise from, for lack of a better word, an "irritation" of the brain.

Depression can cloud one's view of the world with a pervasive negativity laced with fault-finding. Anger can lead to aggressive behavior, possibly with surges of rage. Often one is aware that acting out due to rage is not an acceptable option. Instead, one is forced to internalize it without an outlet for release, leading to a build-up of negative energy that leads to intense frustration.

Perhaps, worse than feeling negative about everything and everyone, is feeling negative about oneself coupled with a severe lack of self-esteem. There is self-blame for perceived weaknesses. One doesn't believe that self-blame is a symptom of the disease if told otherwise. Rather, there is self-loathing with potential for self-harm.

Depression can manifest with a volatility of mood and thought. Psychiatrists often prescribe anti-seizure drugs like Lamictal, Tegretol and Depakote to stabilize the volatile thought patterns of patients with mood disorders. Although my own speculation, it is interesting that the same medications that control the seizure-related spread of uncontrolled neural impulses throughout the brain can also control the spread of neural impulses that cause huge fluctuations of mood and the flood of unwanted, disturbing thoughts that often come at a breakneck pace. Those thoughts can generalize into a global feeling of hopelessness. Hopelessness can become despair. Despair can become paralysis. The paralysis that is part of depression prevents one from being productive or taking any positive steps toward self-care. Often, one cannot muster enough energy to accomplish the simplest of tasks. For many, getting out of bed is too onerous.

Depression not only affects mood, but also can cause cognitive difficulties, including deceased concentration and memory. Completing projects is difficult, but even more so, starting them can be a challenge. One may lack any desire to participate in group activities or interact with anyone, in part ascribed to a feeling of generalized fatigue.

Another prominent component of depression is generalized anxiety. Of course, anxiety disorders need not be associated with depression. Anxiety is a manifestation of feeling unsafe or out of control. Depression has the power to elicit both. The close companion of anxiety is irritability. Irritability is also a close relative of rage and anger.

Depression-related physiologic changes include a change in appetite and sleep disturbances. With regard to the former, weight loss or weight gain can occur with depression. Anxiety can result from the knowledge that a particular anti-depressant medication you are taking has a propensity to promote weight gain. A craving for carbs and a need to stress eat that seems out of one's control can worsen anxiety.

With regard to sleep disturbances, insomnia can manifest

as a difficulty initiating sleep or staying asleep, including early morning awakening. With the latter, one awakens in the early morning hours, such as two or three o'clock, with trouble returning back to sleep. Interestingly, alcohol, which is a depressant, can produce the same exact sleep disturbance if large enough quantities are imbibed. Similarly, the depressant effects of alcohol can make some people quite angry. In contradistinction to early morning awakening, some people experience a difficulty initiating sleep. Awareness of disturbing thoughts are often worse at bedtime. One lies in bed in a dark, quiet room, but does not experience the inner quiet necessary to induce sleep. Rather, one is alone with mind chatter, rumination and anxiety often centered around the possibility of being exhausted the next day as the time ticks onward. Alternatively, depression can cause hypersomnia, or increased sleepiness, and excessive daytime somnolence.

Of course, suicidal ideations often occur in depressed individuals. It is paradoxical that a primal motivating force of the human species is survival, yet the psychic pain and suffering of depression can force one to desire just the opposite. It is a well-known phenomenon that many patients with depression often commit suicide, not when they are in deep depressions, but rather after pharmacological intervention that allows the paralysis to abate just enough to turn ideations into a suicide attempt.

It bears repeating or if you happened to skip over the introduction, as I often do when I read books:

If at this time, you find yourself in a dark place, please reach out to loved ones, friends, professionals or others for support. I have been in that dark place and I can assure you that eventually the psychic pain resolves and feelings of desperation abate. A suicide attempt is often a cry for help. Before you get to that point, make sure you cry out loudly to all of those that can help you. They are depending on you!

<u>Dialing 988</u> is a direct link to:
> the National Suicide Prevention Hotline
> https://suicidepreventionlifeline.org.

You will be able to talk to a caring, nonjudgmental person.

As you probably can tell from my aforementioned description, depression is a daily struggle. There is a formal definition of clinical depression put forth in the Diagnostic and Statistical Manual of Mental Disorders or DSM-5, formulated by the American Psychiatric Association. The most prevalent manifestation of clinical depression is major depressive disorder. At times, the American Psychiatric Association refers to depression and anxiety as "disorders" rather than "diseases" or "illnesses" in describing clinical depression and anxiety. The root "dis" means "not", such that "disorder" literally means "not in order". In a sense, "disorder" implies a state of confusion. I personally don't feel confused or disordered when I experience depression and anxiety. Perhaps, "disorder" is a more euphemistic term and, therefore, carries less of a stigma.

As a radiologist and one who experiences depression and anxiety, I prefer to use what I believe are more accurate descriptors that reflect my medical sensibilities and are more consistent with my own experience. Therefore, I have taken the liberty throughout this book to refer to depression and anxiety as "mental disease" or "mental illness", rather than "mental disorders." In medicine, when there is any structural or functional abnormality affecting a particular organ, we consider it a disease, whether genetic or acquired, such as heart disease or liver disease. In essence, depression and anxiety can be considered diseases of the brain, whether genetic or acquired, as there is a dysfunction of the system of neurotransmitters responsible for mood, as well as structural abnormalities found in the anatomy of the brain, including portions of the amygdala, hippocampus, thalamus and cerebral cortex. In addition, the root "dis" means "not" and one definition of "ease" is a feeling of comfort, such that "disease" literally means "not comfortable". "Illness" is the state of being unhealthy. I can assure you that depression and anxiety make me both uncomfortable and feel unhealthy. Along with symptoms reflecting alterations in mood and mentation, there are also many physical symptoms that comprise depression and anxiety. Symptoms are manifestations of disease states, so that despite the trend towards using "disorder" rather than "disease" or "illness", I prefer to state that I have a mental disease or mental illness.

Nonetheless, according to the DSM-5, specific criteria for major depressive disorder include at least five of the following symptoms that are present, typically most of the day and nearly everyday, during the same two week period, with at least one of those symptoms being anhedonia, or diminished interest and/or pleasure, or depressed mood.

Possible symptoms of major depressive disorder include:

- depressed mood
- anhedonia - diminished interest or pleasure in all, or almost all, activities
- significant weight loss when not dieting or weight gain or decrease or increase in appetite
- sleep disturbance - insomnia or hypersomnia
- psychomotor agitation or retardation
- fatigue or loss of energy
- feelings of worthlessness or excessive or inappropriate guilt
- diminished ability to think or concentrate
- recurrent thoughts of death, recurrent suicidal ideation without a specific plan, a suicide attempt or a specific plan for committing suicide

For some, these symptoms are quite visible to others. Many with a diagnosis of depression, however, have developed the ability to hide their suffering and psychic pain. I have learned that you never know who those people might be. I, for one, had a successful career as a radiologist for thirty years and no one knew of my diagnosis.

Apropos to the idea of the ability to hide one's suffering from others are lyrics to the song by Amandla Stenberg, Benj Pasek and Justin Paul, *The Anonymous Ones*, from the movie version of *Dear Evan Hansen,* a moving Broadway musical dealing with themes of mental illness and suicide.

You ever looked at all the people
    Who seem to know exactly how to be
    You think, "They don't need piles of prescriptions
    To function naturally"

Well, look again, and you might catch it
    Just stay a minute more
    There's this little moment after the sunny smile
    As their eyes fall to the floor

And the truth starts peaking through
    They're a lot like me and you
    They can fake a smile too

The anonymous ones

    Never let you see the ache they carry

    All of those anonymous ones

    Who never name the quiet pain they bury

    So they keep on keeping secrets that

    they think they have to hide

    But what if everybody's secret is they have that secret side?

    And to know they're somehow not alone

    Well, that's all they're hoping for

    What if they didn't have to stay

    Anonymous anymore?

Spot the girl who stays in motion

    She spins so fast so she won't fall

    She's built a wall with her achievements

    To keep out the question

    "Without it, is she worth anything at all?"

    So nobody can know

    Just what the cracks might show

    How deep and dark they go

They are those anonymous ones

    Stuck inside the perfect frame they're faking

    All of us anonymous ones

    Who pick themselves apart 'til they start breaking

    And we keep on keeping secrets that

    we think we have to hide

But what we really need is somebody

to see that secret side

And to know we're somehow not alone

Is all we're hoping for

And that we wouldn't have to be

Anonymous anymore

The parts we can't tell, we carry them well

But that doesn't mean they're not heavy

The parts we can't tell, we carry them well

But that doesn't mean they're not heavy

The anonymous one

Noticed by none

The parts we can't tell, we carry them well

But that doesn't mean they're not heavy

The parts we can't tell

We carry them well

But that doesn't mean they're not heavy

The parts we can't tell

We carry them well

But that doesn't mean they're not heavy

The anonymous ones

Might just need this moment to remind them

That there are more anonymous ones

They're out there if you take the time to find them

Just to know we're somehow not alone

Isn't that all we're ever really looking for?

Maybe we

We don't have to be

Anonymous anymore

The point is, that for some their disease is visible, but for many others, they choose and are able to keep it hidden. Although representing my own speculation based on personal experience, I believe that a higher level of daily functioning relates to greater resiliency, not to the degree of one's suffering. That resiliency allowed me to overcome my intense psychic pain that enabled me to realize professional success, however, without a lessening of the intensity of suffering related to my depression. But, just like an anonymous one, my isolation with my disease worsened my symptoms without the luxury of interacting with like-minded people.

The song also addresses the need for many with mental illness to keep it hidden lest they risk ridicule by others whom are ignorant and propagate the stigma of mental illness. As a yoga instructor, I am gentle with all my students, since I can never really know who suffers from mental disease and/or past traumas. In my case, I felt exposing my mental disease to medical colleagues would be professional suicide. The stigma of mental illness continues to persist, even in the medical profession. Now that I have moved on to my second career as yoga instructor and author, I have the liberty to freely discuss my mental challenges. Even more so, it is so very important for me to do so in hope that we can get closer to the expression of common decency and respect that everyone deserves, regardless of whatever challenge they might face. Quite simply, I no longer need to be anonymous any more.

Situational depression is any of the aforementioned symptoms of clinical depression brought about by a traumatic life event, such as loss of a loved one. Situational depression might be short-lived or potentially last for months or even years. Situational depression can be layered upon clinical depression. Once again my own speculation, as I cannot speak of others' experiences, but I believe that the magnitude of psychic pain is unrelated to whether depression might be clinical or situational.

Anxiety disorders can also be clinical or situational. Rather than normal feelings of nervousness related to an external stressor, anxiety is considered abnormal when it is disproportionate to the level of stress one is experiencing. At its worst, it can be disabling and paralyzing, interfering with normal functioning. Specific clinical anxiety disorders include phobias, generalized anxiety disorder, and panic disorder. Post-traumatic stress disorder or PTSD can manifest in any of the above forms. A friend of mine did two tours of duty in Afghanistan. For him, flying on an airplane can serve as a trigger that brings him emotionally back to the battlefield. I have my own battles with PTSD, as I was subject to both verbal and sexual abuse as a child and teenager. My PTSD manifest as occasional panic attacks laced with a racing heart, perspiration and an adrenalin rush that is telling my body to run away from the source of abuse, albeit just a memory.

The autonomic nervous system governs the physical symptoms of anxiety. The sympathetic component or the "flight or fight" response is activated by conscious perception of being unsafe or out of control. Pulse rate, blood pressure and respiratory rate increase and blood is diverted away from non-vital organs, such as the digestive track. I will further explore this physiological response to stress in greater detail in a subsequent chapter on the body-mind connection. Suffice it to say now, the sympathetic response is a healthy one in the face of actual danger, as it provides the necessary physiologic changes to assure survival. It becomes unhealthy when it continues to initiate those changes in chronic anxiety disorders, when one's mortality is not threatened.

Chronic depression and anxiety can also be related to habitual, automatic, negative thoughts that manifest as cognitive distortions. Being mired in pervasive negativity interferes with a healthy outlook and the experience of contentment and peace. Common cognitive distortions that can be obstacles to developing a healthy outlook, and in the context of this book, the proper mindset to practice yoga, include negative self-judgments arising from comparison to others based in a poor self-image, magnifying the negative aspects of a situation by filtering out the positives, dismissing any possibility of success through polarized or black or white thinking, and presuming to know what others are thinking, assuming that their thoughts cast you in a negative light. I will also delve further into cognitive distortions in a subsequent chapter on a healthier mind. Suffice it to say now, possibilities for distorting one's reality to support feelings of low self-esteem unfortunately abound.

Substitution of positive affirmations for automatic negative thoughts can result in significant stress reduction. Thoughts of gratitude and appreciation might be substituted for negative self-judgments. Just like negative thought patterns, newfound positive ones can also become habitual. Once that occurs, you are on the road to some peace of mind, increased self-esteem, and self-satisfaction. Of course, this is all easier said than done since our reflexive negative thoughts and behaviors are ingrained defense mechanisms that have been reinforced over many years. Similar to becoming more flexible both mentally and physically through yoga, a change in mindset occurs gradually and requires patience. Small "baby steps" can promote feelings of accomplishment that promote a positive outlook and create momentum towards productive change and personal growth.

Stress, one target of yoga, fuels both depression and anxiety. It represents an even more amorphous concept than those of depression or anxiety. One definition from the Oxford Languages is, "a state of mental or emotional strain or tension resulting from adverse or very demanding circumstances." The experience of stress is a universal one, whether it be from work, relationships, time constraints, or finances, to name just a few on a very long list. There are both internal and external stressors. Internal stressors are most often the result of the interpretation of and the response to external stressors. The hope is that learned relaxation through a regular yoga practice will mute the internal stress responses to external stressors, while at the same time effect long term beneficial changes on the physical body and its functioning.

Mental diseases manifest in many different forms. Their commonality lies in the psychic pain that they all cause. The experience of psychic pain is beyond description. It might be analogous to attempting to describe in words how vanilla ice cream tastes or how the color red looks without using the words vanilla or red. The unbearable physical pain from touching a scalding hot pot or an accidental laceration with a kitchen knife are easy to understand. Unfortunately, most of us can relate to the experience of physical pain, perceived by the brain as secondary to an injury to the physical body. That physical pain may be short-lived or possibly more chronic, but we can all relate to the experience. Psychic pain is beyond description. For me, psychic pain is worse than any physical pain I can experience, made worse by the dreadful feeling that it is unrelenting and without end. Anesthetics, analgesics and anti-inflammatories can all treat physical pain. Psychic pain can seem inescapable with no direct or immediate form of relief. It is certainly my own speculation, but I believe that, for some, self-harm is a way of substituting physical pain for psychic pain, the former seemingly more tolerable with its etiology fully known and understandable.

Finally, the aforementioned discussion is quite basic. Mental disease is an extremely complex subject with enumerable nuances on which dedicated books and treatises have been written. Although I have segregated mental diseases into separate entities, they can all be intertwined into a global disease process that presses down upon the spirit. They are diseases that are not well understood, although medical research is slowly uncovering their etiologies and abnormal physiology.

I believe if there is one benefit of having mental struggles, it is possessing greater empathy for others that suffer. If you are facing difficult mental challenges that interfere with your enjoyment of life, my heart truly goes out to you. I try to offer support with my words that are an attempt to describe yoga as a unique coping mechanism in the form of a spiritually-uplifting practice. I have been able to better cope with my mental challenges by reaping all of the benefits that yoga has to offer. I sincerely wish to offer you a similar opportunity. It is my hope that you will embrace yoga and find solace, contentment and peace of mind. Allow your yoga to be an opportunity for self-discovery with the important realization that mental disease does not define you. It is what you have, not who you are!

3

WHAT IS RELAXATION AND HOW TO ACHIEVE IT

A ccording to Oxford Languages, definitions of the word, "relaxation" include:

- the state of being free from tension and anxiety
- recreation or rest, especially after a period of work
- the loss of tension in a part of the body, especially in a muscle when it ceases to contract
- the action of making a rule or restriction less strict
- the restoration of equilibrium following a disturbance

I will consider each of these definitions separately. They are all applicable to the practice of yoga and embody the art of relaxation. Just as one word can have multiple meanings, yoga can open our minds to so many varied novel perspectives that can foster personal growth and wellbeing.

---

1) The state of being free from tension and anxiety

Tension and anxiety are manifestations of feeling unsafe or out of control. When faced with an immediate danger, these emotions are important coping mechanisms, sometimes life-saving. When anxiety and stress become chronic and generalized, they become unhealthy to both the body and spirit. Regrets of the past may stem from perceived wrong decisions and bad choices, some of which might have seemed out of one's control. Reliving past traumas can return one to a time when they felt unsafe. Similarly, concerns about the future can be anxiety-provoking. Predicting failure or disaster that seems to be out of one's control elicits feelings of fear and dread. Often those predictions can be self-fulfilling prophecies. A corollary of predicting the future is superstitiousness; a compulsion to consider the worst possible outcome to a future event lest it will occur. This distorted manner of thinking is reinforced by the low probability that a disastrous outcome will ever occur. Worrying to avert a plane crash is reinforced by the unlikely possibility of one. A close relative of superstitiousness is magical thinking; believing that one has the power through their behavior or actions to alter future events, such as believing that a positive outcome to a sporting event is predicated on wearing a certain team jersey or T-shirt.

In the setting of chronic depression and generalized anxiety, rumination on past and potential future disease-related suffering that seems out of one's control can result in incapacitating stress and a paralysis that prevents any attempt at self-care, including practicing yoga. In addition, the suffering and psychic pain of depression and anxiety can become the focus of mind chatter, especially the feelings of hopelessness from an expectation that neither will ever improve.

It is much more easier said than done, but a de-emphasis of those negative thoughts is accomplished by living in the present moment. Focusing on what is happening in the present blocks the brain from generating thoughts about the past or future. Although millions of impulses and signals are generated by the brain each minute, one might postulate that the mind can only handle one conscious thought at a time. Our goal is to create a string of thoughts that keeps us in the present and away from the past or future. The power of yoga to relax lies in the ability to generate an idea or thought that is concerned with what is occurring at any given moment, which as alluded to in the first chapter can be realized through the practice of mindfulness. I will discuss mindfulness in greater detail in a subsequent chapter. Suffice it to say, mindfulness is experiencing the present moment by engaging the fives senses: touch, sight, hearing, smell and taste. As you will read later on, I add the additional "internal" senses of stretch and proprioception, or the position of the body in space, and the sense of insight. Although on the face of it, it seems that we are focusing on a particular physical sensation, in actuality we are focusing on the thought that is created by the brain's interpretation of that physical sensation. As such, we can focus on any thought that is concerned with what we are doing at a given moment. Those thoughts can come from personal meanings or novel ideas from knowledge of yogic philosophy, human physiology and science that pertain to a particular pose or a breathing technique in which we are engaged.

---

2) Relaxation as recreation or rest, especially after a period of work

Although this definition of relaxation seems to be one that shouldn't require too much explanation or analysis, it possesses many nuances, especially as they pertain to the practice of yoga. Resting might be defined as an opportunity to lessen or eliminate external stressors, which is consistent with the aforementioned first definition of relaxation, that of freedom from tension and anxiety. Resting could also be considered taking a break from work, the consequent stress reduction from which becomes even greater by layering on pleasurable, recreational activities. Recreation can be invigorating and restorative, as well.

Yoga can be considered one form of recreation. One

heteronym of the word "recreate" means to create again. In a sense, through yoga, we are regenerating energy that has been depleted by the stresses of life, which manifests as greater resiliency. Of course, relaxation is not particular to yoga. We could also define recreation as any pleasurable activity that has the power to relax. In the practice of yoga, there are many sources of pleasure, including the stretching of muscles, interacting with like-minded people in a yoga class, experiencing the collective energy of the *sangha,* or community, and breathing deeply to induce waves of relaxation, to name just a few.

Relaxation is best experienced in times of rest between the *asanas.* As it bears repeating, "the magic of yoga occurs in the spaces between the postures," when activity transitions into stillness. From a physical perspective, which on the face of it may not seem that magical, muscles function better when given time to recover from use. Oxygen can better nourish overworked muscles during periods of rest. Rest after activity allows the core temperature of the body to return to baseline. From a spiritual point of view, a period of stillness is an opportunity to better connect with oneself by digesting the emotional effects of an active physical body on the mind.

In yoga, as in life, we always strive for balance. Yoga is about creating a good balance between activity and rest. Spiritually, we try to internalize and balance *prana,* the life force in the universe that surrounds us all. The breath is the vehicle to bring *prana* inward. Once taken into the body, it must then be balanced throughout all of the energy pathways. Balance in yoga comes in many different forms. One might imagine deeply inhaling the positive energy of *prana* and ridding the body of negativity and mental waste known as *apana* with each exhalation. Whether positive energy is experienced spiritually or physically, it is balance in life that is a stabilizing force. With stability come feelings of safety and control. Once we no longer feel unsafe or out of control, relaxation ensues.

---

3) The loss of tension in a part of the body, especially in a muscle when it ceases to contract

Muscles have two states: contraction and relaxation. Antagonistic muscles exist throughout the body. Antagonistic muscles don't hate each other or fight with one another. Rather, they have opposite, yet complimentary functions. For example, the biceps and triceps in the upper arm are antagonistic. Contraction of the biceps muscle flexes the arm while the triceps is passively stretched. Contraction of the triceps muscle extends the arm out straight while the biceps is passively stretched. You can feel this effect by placing your hand on the biceps as you flex and extend the arm. The muscle will contract and release with the movement. Various muscle groups have opposing functions. The inner thigh muscles or hip adductors are antagonistic to the hip abductors, the former pulling the thighs together with contraction and the latter pulling them apart and rotating the hips out laterally as they contract. Once again, when the adductors contract, the abductors passively stretch, and vice versa. Similarly, muscles along one side of the forearm extend the wrist and fingers and are antagonistic to muscles on the other side that result in flexion. In all of the warm-ups and *asanas* we assume throughout our practice, antagonistic muscles are constantly working and releasing as we move. These actions allow the muscles to have periods of active contraction and passive stretching, or more simply, work and rest. Periods of release and relaxation of the muscles protect them from overuse and potential tears and assure a more than adequate delivery of oxygen to the muscle fibers.

Over time, this interplay of antagonistic muscles results in an increase in strength and flexibility. Contraction strengthens and relaxation allows for stretching and an increase in flexibility. As we assume pose and counterpose, alternating energy flows from one muscle group to another. One pose-counterpose combination often done in yoga is the cat and cow poses. As we assume the cow, the tailbone rises, the back arches and the chest and gaze lift. These movements reverse in the cat as the back rounds, the chest drops, gaze is directed at the knees and the tailbone is tucked in. The alternating arching and rounding of the back are complex movements involving numerous muscle groups of the core. Some muscles contract to arch the back. As the back rounds, those same muscles relax and stretch and the corresponding antagonistic muscles contract. By having a heightened focus on the action of the body in any pose and counterpose, the brain is learning the sensations of muscular tension and release. Learned relaxation includes achieving a conscious awareness of that release, accessing it at any time in order to physically relax. As an example, many of us carry our tension in the muscles of the neck and shoulders. We are often unaware that we are chronically shrugging our shoulders. As an exercise, as you take a deep inhalation, consciously shrug your shoulders toward the ears. As you slowly exhale, let the shoulder blades melt down the back as you experience muscular release in the neck and shoulders. Habits are difficult to break, but practicing this exercise periodically throughout a busy, stressful day will go a long way in making a relaxed state of the neck and shoulder muscles the norm.

Returning back to the definition of relaxation as a loss of tension in part of the body, ultimately mastering a conscious awareness of muscular relaxation results in a decrease in mental tension. Herein lies the body-mind connection. They are inseparable. The mind directs the body and the state of the body affects the mind as it reacts to physical sensations with thoughts and emotions. When the sensations arise from physical relaxation, the mind experiences feelings of pleasure, relief and release.

4) The action of making a rule or restriction less strict

I will first consider rules and then restrictions. With regard to yoga, there is only one rule: to make your practice your own personal experience while practicing self-observation without judgment. As you participate in a yoga class, it seems that numerous rules exist for the ideal performance of a particular *asana,* or pose. In some classes, the instructor can become the enforcer of those rules by offering individual corrections or assists, either verbal or hands-on. Self-judgments are unavoidable if someone is corrected while assuming a particular *asana.* Inherently, the person being corrected assumes that what he, she or they is doing is wrong. The person on the adjacent mat that is not being corrected assumes that he, she or they is doing it right. Even if these corrections are welcomed, the flooding of the mind with thoughts of a need to perform the posture according to the "rules" is unavoidable. These thoughts don't serve us and are antithetical to the goal of gaining mental clarity. If unwelcome, corrections can further cloud the mind with negative self-judgments and self-consciousness. Always remember that the *asanas* were created to serve as a consistent way to communicate one form or tradition of yoga from person to person or class to class. Rather than concerning yourself with performing all of the postures perfectly, make them your own expression. Enjoy your unique movements and then enhance that enjoyment by connecting them to the breath.

Let's consider the accepted way to ideally assume *Matsyen-*

drasana, the Lord of the Fishes pose or the seated spinal twist. In practice, an instructor offers cues to guide students into the poses. For the purposes of this discussion, however, we can substitute the word, "rule", for the word, "cue".

The following are all the "rules" for assuming the ideal version of *Matsyendrasana:*

1. The inside edge of one foot, let us say the left foot, is placed on the inside of the right thigh.
2. Option to place the left foot on the outside of the right thigh.
3. The right hand holds on to the bent left knee or the inside of the right elbow wraps around the knee.
4. The left hand is positioned on the mat behind and close to the back.
5. The spine is twisted to the left.
6. Gaze is over the left shoulder.
7. The heel of the extended right leg is pushed away from the body to stretch the muscles along the back of the leg, including the hamstrings.
8. The back should not be rounded. The spine should be as long and straight as possible. This is facilitated three ways: 1) with each inhalation, pulling the left thigh towards the belly to elongate the spine. 2) by moving the left hand as close to the back as possible and 3) sitting on the edge of a bolster or cushion.

9. The spine and back should be perfectly straight.

10. With each inhalation, one attempts to lengthen the torso more and more. With each exhalation, one attempts to twist the spine more and more.

11. Although diaphragmatic breathing is limited with a twisted torso, breathe as deeply as possible.

12. In the full expression of this pose, tension exists throughout the body. The ultimate goal is to divert the mind from physical tension to feelings of inwardness by bringing all of your awareness to the breath.

This certainly sounds like a lot of rules. A dedication to those rules diverts the mind from other more important thoughts.

For example, if you have limited ability to twist relating to neck or back discomfort or one's body habitus, potential lamentations over not being able to "do" the posture as everyone else may arise. Thoughts that are laced with physical and/or mental stress become your focus.

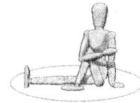

Matsyendrasana ~ The Lord of the Fishes Pose or The Seated Spinal Twist

We need to choose an intention when performing *Matsyendrasana* that promotes single-pointed concentration and relaxation and then dedicate our thoughts to that intention. My intention may be different than yours. My intention often changes each time I assume the pose. At times, I choose to focus on the breath, listening to each inhalation as my spine "grows" in length and each exhalation as I twist a little more each time. Sometimes, my intention is to observe physical sensations using the practice of mindfulness. Using the sense of touch, I can appreciate the contact points of my body on the mat or the feeling of my hand or elbow on my knee. As I gaze over my shoulder, I use the sense of vision to notice what lies behind me, an action I often do not do. I might become aware of the physicality of the pose, breathing into the spinal twist, or scanning the body, noticing which muscles are tense and contracted and those that are passively stretched. While assuming *Matsyendrasana*, I often consider the symbolism and meaning of the story of Matysendranath, a sage and author who lived in the 10th century, CE, credited with founding Hatha yoga and the namesake of this pose. He is an important figure in Hinduism. His name literally translates to "Lord of the Fishes". According to Hindu mythology, Matsyendranath was swallowed by a fish after his parents, fearful of the omen of an ill-fated star, tossed their baby into the ocean. One day, the fish swam to the seabed where Matysendranath overheard the god Shiva revealing the secrets of Hatha yoga to Parvati, the Hindu goddess of fertility, beauty and love. In possession of those secrets, Matysendranath practiced yoga in the belly of the fish for many years, ultimately emerging as a spiritually aware yogi, and ultimately the Lord of the Fishes. The many meanings that lie in this story include striving for personal growth through a disciplined practice despite a situation that could cause one to despair. This sentiment is quite analogous to the plight of those with mental illness. Rather than giving in to despair in the face of psychic pain and suffering, it is possible to undergo a personal transformation through a dedication to the practice of yoga. Finally, while reflecting on the story of Matysendraneth, I can also pay homage to this ancient practice of yoga and its origins that date back centuries.

Whatever your intention might be, being true to that intention requires dismissing any compulsion to perform the posture perfectly. Perfection in yoga and in life is an unrealistic expectation. Part of achieving relaxation is freeing oneself from rules, especially those that are self-imposed. As is true in life, it is healthier not to be the one that enforces those rules by constantly correcting yourself.

With regard to the easing of restrictions as a definition for relaxation, yoga is a vehicle for removing any restraints that press down upon the spirit. Freeing yourself from self-imposed restrictions as you practice yoga brings clarity of mind, with the potential for connecting with one's true authenticate self. It is gaining awareness of how you wish to live, rather than living restricted by someone else's expectations of who they think you should be. Often during childhood, expectations for how we should behave are set by our parents, along with the influence of societal norms. Unfortunately for many, those expectations aren't consistent with their true desire as how they wish to live. Often, as if they are attempting to mold their children according to their own life expectations, parents impose restrictions on the expression of the child's own desires. A healthier scenario is allowing the child to explore, find their passion and live life governed by their own goals and desires. These inconsistencies between parental expectations and a child's desires cause inner conflicts that can persist into adulthood, often manifest as dysphoria that fuels depression and anxiety.

Dysphoria is a discontent that develops secondary to restrictions placed on often repressed deep-rooted thoughts and desires. If we define it as a discontent that arises from an inconsistency of one's reality and one's true passions, dysphoria could be secondary to conflicts arising from sexual or gender identity, but also from poor career choices, dysfunctional relationships or anything else that is inconsistent with one's true authentic self.

In our present day, dysphoria most commonly refers to a state of unhappiness or discomfort relating to an inconsistency of gender identity and biological sex assigned at birth. Gender identity is a complex subject with many defined classifications, including cisgender, transgender, non-binary, gender queer and gender fluid. There is a very broad spectrum of gender identities, ranging from transgender to cisgender, and, as such, specific labels aren't necessarily applicable to each individual person. Each one of us lies somewhere on that spectrum, the exact location of which may be fluid on different days or at different times of life. Gender identity is not an absolute, black and white issue. It is not a binary expression of either wishing to be a man or woman, but rather, a nuanced, individual non-binary one where masculine and feminine desires differ in degrees of expression.

Gender dysphoria can be the cause of depression and anxiety or add to the symptoms of preexisting clinical disease. It is sometimes lessened by activities and dress that conform to one's perceived gender in a cultural context. Societal norms determine what are considered masculine and feminine behaviors. Many times those norms are arbitrary. The makeup, wigs and dress worn in the royal court of King Louis XIV would be considered quite feminine by today's standards. Many present cultures openly accept transgender and gender fluid individuals. The Fa'afafines and Fa'afatamas of traditional Samoan culture are names that describe gender fluid people that were assigned male and female at birth, respectively. The Sakalava people of Madagascar recognize a third gender comprised of boys who exhibit feminine behaviors and are subsequently raised as girls. Many native North American peoples revere transgender individuals, calling them "two-spirit"; possessing both female and male spirits. There are many other examples of cultures throughout the world that embrace various gender identities. In those societies, presumably there is a relative absence of gender dysphoria. Traditionally, in our Western society, boys play with trucks and toy guns and girls with dolls and tea sets. These behaviors are also cultural. Cultural norms can be fluid, however, as evinced by a trend toward more gender neutral toys and play.

Although nonconforming behaviors can lessen gender dysphoria, doing so can result in other untoward sources of stress, which also can be a source of depression and anxiety. These include intolerance by others resulting in ridicule or bullying. Lack of understanding by a significant other can lead to feelings of being judged with consequent lowered self-esteem. Radical shifts in behaviors and outward expression can also lead to a loss of relationships with family and friends. These external stressors likely contribute to the extremely disproportionate suicide rate and rate of suicide attempts seen in the transgender population.

We can consider the gender spectrum in the context of yogic philosophic principles that advance that we all possess both feminine and masculine energies. Spiritually, we strive for a balance between the complementry energies of the *ida* and *pingala nadis*. *Nadis* are energy channels analogous to the extensive network of nerves that course throughout the body. *Prana*, the life force that surrounds us all, once taken in, flows throughout the body through the *nadis*. Through yoga, we strive to balance *prana* within our physical and spiritual selves. Depending on the particular source cited, it is felt that there are anywhere from 72,000 to 350,000 or possibly even millions of *nadis* in the human body.

The *ida* and *pingala nadis* are two of the main energy channels that criss-cross the spine, intersecting at each of the *chakras,* or main energy centers. They originate at the root or *muladhara chakra* and channel energy superiorly, terminating at the left and right nostril, respectively. When we are active, we experience the energy of the *pingala nadi*, which is felt to be masculine, heat-producing, irrational, impulsive and extroverted, but at the same time fueling strength and vitality in body and mind. During periods of rest, we can harness the energy of the *ida nadi*, which is feminine, cool, rational, insightful and introverted. As one is cool and one is hot, the *ida* and *pingala nadis* are also referred to as the moon and sun channels, respectively.

As previously mentioned, a goal of yoga is establishing balance, in this case between the feminine energy of the *ida nadi* and the masculine energy of the *pingala nadi*. Accessing the active, irrational and impulsive energy of the *pingala* can stir up repressed emotions and thoughts. At the same time, tapping into the rational and analytical energy of the *ida* allows us to witness that which has been exposed. Witnessing repressed emotions can be anxiety-provoking, but liberating at the same time, releasing one from inner conflict through understanding, awareness and acceptance. By applying the concept of the energies of the *ida* and *pingala*, one's place on the gender spectrum might be considered a perception of one's more dominant qualities, being either more feminine or masculine, expressed in either conformity or nonconformity with societal norms. That perception may be fluid; the relative strengths and dominance of the *ida* and *pingala nadis* varying over time.

The process of exposing and witnessing deep-rooted thoughts and emotions can lead to the discovery of one's true authentic self. In order for that discovery to be liberating, it need not lead to radical changes in lifestyle or behaviors. The easing of dysphoria-related depression and anxiety isn't necessarily dependent on nonconformity from societal norms, since ultimately those norms are arbitrary. The yogic philosophical idea of the existence of both fluid feminine and masculine energies within each and everyone of us that are expressed to different degrees at different times is a healthier way to consider gender identity. Even more so, perhaps those that balance their female and male energies have the luxury of tapping into both, enjoying all that life has to offer with freedom of thought and behavior. Yoga fosters an ability for outward self-expression of ideas and emotions. Expressions of love, compassion and gratitude, developing physical strength and tapping into one's grace through the fluidity of movement need not be and should not be gender specific.

Unfortunately, the female gender stereotype of the practitioner of yoga is so pervasive in Western culture, advanced by online and print content that is targeted at women, including advertisements for everything from women's clothing to feminine hygiene products. In many yoga magazines, most of the models in photos demonstrating the *asanas* are women. Yoga is a multibillion dollar business in the United States, including hundreds of millions of dollars spent on advertising. The retail business of yoga, including the sales of designer leggings, is flourishing. Yoga as a business can be at odds with yoga as a spiritual practice.

Because of the marketing of yoga in the Western world, many men consider yoga to be a feminine pursuit. Many men would prefer to not think of being the only male in a yoga class surrounded by women in spandex leggings. During conversations about my newfound discovery of the benefits of yoga and my enjoyment of my daily practice, the first question asked by both my mother and many of my friends was, "Are you the only man in the class?" Of course, the definition of "manly" should include self-confidence and pride resulting from taking steps to improve one's physical and mental health and establishing a profound dedication to a receptive attitude, which I can assure you the practice of yoga affords. Once again, cultural norms are fluid and fortunately it seems there is a trend toward gender inclusivity in yoga classes, especially with the younger generations, which, at least from my observations, are more progressive, open-minded and accepting.

The positive effects of yoga on the physical body are not gender-specific. Strength, flexibility, cardiovascular health, and improved immunity, to name a few, can be enjoyed by anyone. Our culture thrives on distinctions and differences, whether based in wealth, religion, or political affiliation, to name just a few. This is especially true in the attitudes toward those that deviate from societal norms with regard to sexuality and gender. Perhaps, we would have a healthier, more peaceful world if there was more emphasis on our commonalities and less on distinctions and less energy devoted to restrictions and more on freedoms.

Achieving periods of mental clarity during a yoga practice can afford one the opportunity for self-discovery. Once awareness and acceptance are realized, any lifestyle changes needed to ease the dysphoria stemming from career choices, relationships, sexuality or gender can be implemented if felt to be necessary for satisfaction and contentment. Unfortunately, change is difficult and many let inertia keep them in the same life trajectory, no matter how unhealthy it might be. According to Newton's first law of motion, inertia will carry an object in a straight line unless a force is applied upon it. Relaxing any restrictions to change, finding the energy to make change and finding a life trajectory that is more aligned with one's true desires and passions are all facilitated through states of inwardness, mental clarity and self-analysis that are all realized through yoga.

---

5) The restoration of equilibrium following a disturbance

I believe that for most, the symptoms of depression and

anxiety are not constant. They can vary over time. For some with bipolar disorder, one can cycle from depression to mania and back again. The presence of stress, whether external or internal, can drive anxiety and depression, exacerbating symptoms of both. A disturbance, as noted in the above definition for relaxation, is a good descriptor for a stressor. Like a disturbance in the atmosphere that leads to a storm, a disturbance of the mind can cause a maelstrom of emotions. Yoga affords the opportunity for self-reflection. Discovery of the underlying cause of a mental disturbance as a particular stressor positions you in a better place to cope with that stressor. Learned relaxation through yoga can smooth over the disturbance, returning one back to a state of equilibrium of mood, or at least something that approximates an equilibrium. With mental disease, stability of mood is often not obtainable. At the very least, however, the positive benefits of yoga can decrease the magnitude of the fluctuation of symptoms.

From a physical perspective, a disturbance of the body can arise by practicing yoga beyond one's edge. The edge is the point at which discomfort arises. Aside from being a signal for the potential for injury, physical discomfort can flood the mind with uncomfortable thoughts, making it difficult to find clarity. The best way to practice near one's edge while assuming a particular *asana* is to find the point at which discomfort arises and then ease off from it. An effective method for finding your edge is to enter a posture incrementally. Initially, ease into an *asana* possibly one quarter of the way from your edge, then halfway, and then three quarters, making sure to breathe into each increment. Finally, stretch and engage muscles to the point of discomfort. Then quickly ease off just enough to enjoy the stretch. With time, your edge will begin to advance as you achieve greater flexibility.

There are many ways to approach and interpret the concept of relaxation. Relaxation learned through the practice of yoga can diminish the stress that fuels depression and anxiety. With a realized control of mood, a degree of inner peace and a lessening of the consuming inner turmoil inherent to mental disease are possible. Learning to relax is a step along the path of yoga. As you journey along that path, two realizations are necessary. The first is that there is no final destination. Always striving for greater meaning in your practice constantly opens up new avenues for personal growth. An exploration of your yoga filled with symbolism, insight and reflection has the power to create a multitude of new perspectives. The second realization is that everyone is at a different place on their journey. We all have different thoughts, emotions, intentions and personalities shaped by prior experiences. The interpretation and personal importance of the different aspects of yoga will all differ from one practitioner to the next. Most importantly, as you journey into yoga remove any pressure to make something happen and simply enjoy the process.

We will now take the definition of relaxation one step further by exploring the body-mind connection and the physiological responses of the body to stress. Developing an awareness of what is occurring in the physical body in the face of stress is a vital part of learned relaxation.

4

THE BODY-MIND CONNECTION AND RELAXATION

O ne might argue that a knowledge of the physiological responses of the body to stress or those related to relaxation is not necessary to find peace of mind and contentment through yoga. Part of learned relaxation, however, is being in tune with the body, with an awareness of physical changes that are consciously induced by your yoga practice. A balance between mind and body is facilitated by an awareness of the connection of body to mind. A discussion of the science behind relaxation might be expected to be complex and arcane, but it is a necessary one in order to gain control over stress and anxiety through yoga. So, please stick with me here. I will try to guide you through some complex ideas in an understandable and gentle manner.

Before embarking on our exploration of the physiology of relaxation, it would be good to take a step back and marvel at the miracle that is the human body. Unfathomable complexity exists all the way from the microscopic to the macroscopic levels. At the subcellular level, atomic and subatomic particles intimately interact to create stability out of chaos, harnessing energy to overcome entropy, the randomness that exists in the universe. Elements form that combine to give rise to molecules. The various configurations of those molecules are limitless, yet they organize to become the structure of our cells. The number of cells in the human body is estimated to be in the trillions. Each cell contains a central information center, the nucleus, within which are chromosomes that contain the blueprints of life. Each chromosome is composed of genes consisting of beautiful helices of deoxyribonucleic acid (DNA), encoded with the information to ultimately produce proteins. Those proteins dictate the structure of tissues and organs and their specific functions. We all share many commonalities in gene structure, but the millions of variations and arrangements of genes also gives rise to individuality. Our cells organize into various structures, tissues and organs like the brain, heart and liver and become specialized for specific functions in each. Neurons in the brain conduct electrical signals, cardiac muscle cells contract and release to power the pump that delivers blood and precious oxygen throughout the body, hepatocytes filter toxins and produce bile, hair follicles produce keratin and cells in glands of the endocrine system produce hormones that regulate metabolism, digestion, and mood. As they develop, every cell in the body differentiates to perform a specialized function. They all have different roles to play, but also act in concert to sustain us. It is a veritable symphony made up of trillions of different types of instruments that together produce the music of life. And even more miraculous is that the cells in our brain, these neurons that merely function to transmit electrical signals, allow us to think.

Our thoughts occur both on subconscious and conscious levels. Hundreds of functions operate behind the scenes and out of conscious thought to maintain and sustain the body. Under the so-called "radar" are a myriad of physiologic functions that regulate the vital functions of our cardiovascular, pulmonary, endocrine, genitourinary and digestive systems.

On the conscious level, we can analyze, examine, observe and react. The *asanas* are an integral part of yoga. Each posture requires the movement of particular muscles, tendons, ligaments, joints and bones. Those movements begin in the brain as thoughts. Often we are unaware of those thoughts. Each second the brain produces millions of signals that travel down the spinal cord and throughout the musculoskeletal system, instructing and guiding our limbs, torso, neck and head into orchestrated movements. Sensory receptors embedded throughout the muscles, joints and supporting structures react to movement, subsequently sending messages as electrical signals back to the spinal cord and up to the brain where we can react and feel. Every movement begins and ends with a thought.

Our senses also represent an integral part of the entire mind-body experience of yoga. Chemical reactions in the rods and cones of the retina convert light into electrical signals that are sent to the optic cortex in the brain, allowing us to appreciate whatever we see. By closing the eyes as we practice, we can quiet the activity of the optic tracts and lessen visual stimuli. As we listen to the breath coming in and out of the nose, sound waves that strike the eardrum are transmitted through the ossicles or bones in the middle ear. Mechanical energy is then converted to electrical energy as the sound waves initiate chemical reactions in the hair cells of the cochlear in the inner ear. Electrical signals finally stimulate the auditory cortex of the brain, allowing us to appreciate the sounds we hear. Adjacent to the cochlear is the labyrinth of the inner ear that reacts to motion and imbalance, constantly updating the position of the body in space and activating centers in the brain that bring us to states of stability. If a studio uses incense or a diffuser to fill the air with a scent or possibly you are out in nature practicing yoga, your sense of smell will come into play. Molecules arising from the source of an aroma enter the nostrils as we breathe, eventually reaching chemoreceptors in the nose that also generate electrical signals to ultimately activate the olfactory cortex along the frontal lobes of the brain. As we ground our feet into our mats for the standing *asanas,* sensory receptors in the skin send information to the spinal cord and superiorly to the brain so we can appreciate the feelings of touch, as well as security, safety and balance as we connect with the earth. Proprioreceptors, organelles that relay information about the position of the joints, provide us with an awareness of the body as it moves through space.

Similar physiological functions are ubiquitous throughout the animal world. But, what separates us as unique beings is the capacity for conscious, abstract thought. We can interpret and analyze data. Our abstractions can trigger feelings and emotions. And whether you believe in an actual soul or consider it to be just electrical signals arising from the firings of neurons in the brain, it is that inexplicable part of our personalities that allows us to connect with ourselves and embrace life. Nourishing the soul and connecting with your true authentic self can lead to feelings of contentment, satisfaction and, ultimately, peace. That sense of peace begins with the relationships and interactions of atoms that give rise to the function of cells and complexities of the multilevel hierarchy of tissues and organs of the body.

The human body is certainly a miracle. Through our practice of yoga we can honor that miracle. Yoga provides us with the luxury of time to ponder and wonder about all of the miracles of life and nature. We are a part of the beauty of nature. Accessing that beauty within ourselves leads to self-love. With self-love we can then love others. Atoms to love ~ quite the miracle!

Our journey into the physiology of relaxation begins in prehistoric times with our ancient ancestor, the so-called caveman. This is certainly a misnomer since most of our hominid ancestors were nomadic, not cave dwellers. Nonetheless, for this discussion, a cave represents a place of safety. We might infer that if anxiety is a manifestation of feeling unsafe, our caveman is more likely free of stress in his cave, at least from a mortal danger point of view.

Like many of our ancient ancestors, our caveman is a hunter-gatherer. While on the hunt, he is confronted by a hungry saber-toothed tiger. He is faced with a binary decision: to fight or take flight. Regardless of his choice, his body will react in a similar way to promote his survival. Eventually, he will find himself back in the safety of his cave enjoying a cooked meal, a perfect time for his body to rest and digest. Governing these responses of the body to the presence and absence of external stressors is the autonomic nervous system. In general, its functioning is involuntary, operating in the background of consciousness, hence the qualifier autonomic. As we shall see, however, learning to have some voluntary control over the autonomic nervous system is the key to achieving relaxation. The autonomic nervous system consists of two divisions: the sympathetic and parasympathetic nervous systems, or the fight or flight and the rest and digest systems, respectively. .

Returning back to our caveman in the midst of mortal danger, what does he need physically to survive? Quite simply, his muscles must be operating at maximum efficiency. He requires strength and speed whether deciding to stay and fight or take flight. For muscles to function at their optimum level, they will require as much energy as possible in the form of oxygen and glucose, and then be able to process that energy quickly and efficiently. It will be the sympathetic nervous system that will get the job done.

The sight and sound of the saber-toothed tiger floods our caveman's consciousness. The awareness of danger triggers the sympathetic nervous system. Direct action of sympathetic nerve fibers and the sympathetic-mediated secretion of hormones, including epinephrine, norepinephrine and cortisol sets in motion all of the changes in the body's physiology to help our caveman return to safety. In order to maximize oxygen intake to optimize muscle efficiency, we must first optimize breathing capacity through an increase in respiratory rate and a concomitant dilatation of the airways of the lungs, including the bronchi and bronchioles. In the lungs, oxygen is transferred to the bloodstream. In addition, sympathetic inhibition of insulin secretion by the pancreas results in an increase in blood glucose to "feed" the working muscles.

To move as much blood as fast as possible to maximize the delivery of oxygen and glucose to the muscles, heart rate and blood pressure increase, heart contractions become more forceful and blood vessels dilate. Blood is diverted away from the stomach and intestines to slow down digestion in order to divert energy to other, more vital parts of the body. For our caveman, now is not the time to digest his breakfast.

Actively working muscles generate heat. To lessen the rise of the core body temperature, the sympathetic nervous system stimulates perspiration. Evaporative cooling occurs as secretions from the sweat glands that have been warmed by the body evaporate into the air. The skin becomes flushed, as superficial blood vessels also dilate to release additional body heat. The entire process is analogous to the need to increase production in a factory. The machines in the factory are required to work faster with greater efficiency. More fuel is required to power the machines. As the machines work harder, heat is generated, and some type of cooling mechanism is needed to prevent overheating, which can interfere with proper functioning.

By optimizing the functioning of those parts of the body needed in times of danger, the sympathetic nervous system has increased our caveman's odds of survival. Finally, back in the sanctity of his cave, the sights, scents and sounds of peril and mortal danger have abated, and, as you might guess, it is time for him to rest and digest. It is time for the parasympathetic nervous system to engage. The majority of this division of the autonomic nervous system is derived from the vagus nerve, the ninth of the twelve cranial nerves. *Vagus* is Latin for "wandering". The vagus nerve arises from the brainstem and meanders through the body. In a sense, the parasympathetic system reverses all of the changes implemented by the sympathetic nervous system. Respiratory and heart rate and blood pressure decrease. Insulin is released by the pancreas to decrease blood glucose levels, as the immediate need for higher blood sugar levels lessens. More glucose becomes stored in the liver, ready for release during the next tiger attack. Blood is shunted from skeletal muscles and other organs and tissues critical for survival back to the digestive track with a concomitant increase in motility of the stomach and intestines. Our caveman's skin is drier and his body odor is likely less offensive to his cavewife. From a hormonal perspective, levels of epinephrine (adrenalin), norepinephrine and the stress hormone, cortisol, all drop. The caveman is ready to enjoy his family, a nice meal and a cozy, fire-warmed cave.

It is important to note that although appearing opposite in function, the sympathetic and parasympathetic nervous systems are actually complementary. In fact, a healthy homeostasis is achieved by finding a balance between the two. They are always both active in varying degrees according to the situation at hand. The autonomic nervous system is analogous to a scale that gently moves up and down from one side to the other as we move through our day. For our caveman faced with the saber-toothed, the sympathetic side of his scale is dramatically weighed down. His scale returns back to relative balance when mortal danger resolves.

Now, it is time to travel from the prehistoric world into modern day. With regard to present day gender roles, it might be more accurate to refer to our modern day caveman as a caveperson. The modern day cave might be a house or whatever other shelter in which one might live.

Similar to the prehistoric caveman, as he, she or they goes through their day, the modern day caveperson experiences a relative balance between the sympathetic and parasympathetic nervous systems, with variations in the weight on each side of the scale depending on the presence or absence of external stressors. Extreme external stress, such as experiencing a near-miss automobile accident, might be considered analogous to a saber-toothed tiger attack. In both instances, one is faced with mortal danger. Similar sympathetic-mediated responses are triggered, including an increase in blood pressure and respiratory and heart rates, shunting of the blood to skeletal muscles, vasodilitation, sweating and a rush of adrenalin and cortisol. It is the body's attempt at increasing our chances of survival by heightening our reflexes, enabling us to quickly step on the brake or turn the steering wheel to avert potential danger. This is an appropriate, immediate and short-lived response of the sympathetic nervous system. A problem arises when the sympathetic system continues to trigger the fight or flight response when one is not facing a dangerous situation. A chronic sympathetic response that occurs regardless of one's situation is inappropriate on a physiological level, and ultimately unhealthy. The sympathetic side of the scale becomes asymmetrically and significantly weighed down all of the time, regardless of whether one is faced with danger or not. This persistent asymmetry of autonomic balance is known as chronic sympathetic overload; better known as chronic stress. It is a problem affecting so many of us in our present day culture. Lessening that overload in order to create a healthy balance and a state of wellbeing is the target of yoga. Physical relaxation occurs on an autonomic, physiologic level, but it is through conscious thought that the physiology is controlled. Through yoga, we can find a safe space, both mentally and physically, in which to bring our sympathetic and parasympathetic nervous systems into a healthy state of balance.

Most of the time, modern day cavepeople are not faced with immediate, mortal danger. There are numerous sources of everyday stress from issues in the workplace to problematic relationships to traffic jams during a commute. What is perceived as stressful is particular to the individual. We all have different tolerance levels and degrees of resiliency. More important than the type of external stressor one experiences is the magnitude of their response to it. One person's reaction to a personal computer malfunction might be mild and manageable. Another might experience major angst and frustration. Unfortunately, the autonomic nervous system does not distinguish between actual danger and perceived, sometimes irrational fears and misperceptions of stress. The greater the magnitude of one's emotional reaction to an external or internal stressor, the greater the magnitude of the sympathetic response, whether it be a saber-toothed tiger attack or a traffic jam. The subconscious functioning of the autonomic nervous system only interprets what the conscious mind tells it. Like a car alarm that never shuts off, if one's strong, emotional reactions to stress become habitual, the sympathetic nervous system will continue to function as if that saber-toothed tiger never went away.

With chronic stress, we enter into a state of allostatic loading. Allostatic load was a term coined in 1993 by Bruce Sherman McEwen and Eliot Stellar. Allostasis is the process whereby the body responds to stressors in order to regain homeostasis, a healthy state of equilibrium in the body. With allostatic loading, the system becomes overwhelmed, in essence stuck in a sympathetic overload state, leading to a chronic decline in the health of the organs and tissues of the body, a reduction in resiliency, the inability to react to stressors, and the eventual development of disease states. Returning back to the metaphor of the relationship of the two components of the autonomic nervous system as two sides of a scale, sympathetic on one side and parasympathetic on the other, allostatic loading is analogous to a huge weight pressing down on the former. This chronic stress state results in a whole cascade of detrimental physiologic changes, including the activation or deactivation of genes, a continual flood of stress hormones like cortisol and epinephrine into the bloodstream, a rise in inflammatory molecules and a weakening of the body's immune status. These negative effects can promote a multitude of diseases, including atherosclerosis, hypertension, and heart disease, among numerous others.

Our perceptions of stress and our habitual automatic negative thoughts and behaviors elicited by stress initiate and sustain this process of chronic sympathetic overload and a disruption of normal physiologic homeostasis. In essence, we become unhealthy. The question arises as to how those pervasive negative thoughts and behaviors serve the individual. They are, of course, defense mechanisms that offer protection against external stressors. When those thoughts and behaviors become reflexive to all stressors, regardless of import or severity, generalized anxiety ensues. One solution to break that cycle is retraining the brain to develop appropriate and graded responses to stress. A more acute sympathetic response is beneficial when faced with a real danger, but chronic sympathetic overload is not. Our bodies need a homeostasis or balance between sympathetic and parasympathetic processes. It is appropriate for our proverbial caveman to increase his heart and respiratory rate and divert blood to his skeletal muscles when confronted by the ferocious tiger, but not for that sympathetic response to continue while in the safety of his cave.

Yoga is a powerful tool in developing healthy responses to stress, both mentally and physically. Stress can create a susceptibility to disease, as well as worsen pre-existing disease states. It can also decrease tolerance to the symptoms of depression and anxiety, as well as lessen resiliency that can interfere with daily functioning and an enjoyment of life.

If chronic sympathetic overload is the problem, eliminating chronic stress is the solution. Can we actually have control over physiological processes that are autonomic, involuntary and occurring under the radar? Since these processes occur in the physical body, by connecting the mind to the body, awareness of and eventual control over those processes ensue. As the autonomic nervous system reacts to stressors regardless of origin and with a magnitude related to how the brain interprets the danger associated with a stressor, it is important to habituate to consistently telling the sympathetic nervous system accurate information. The conscious brain must tell the sympathetic nervous system that a computer glitch is merely a nuisance not a mortal attack. A computer glitch does not require the fight or flight response. We need not fight with or run away from our computer. A healthier and more measured response requires neither. The end result is a healthier body and a healthier mind.

Through our practice of yoga, with patience and gradually over time, we can learn to gain voluntary control over the autonomic nervous system by introducing relaxation techniques to achieve appropriate, healthier responses to the stresses of life. We can enjoy a sense of wellbeing centered in a healthy balance of mind and body. There exists an interplay between the body and mind, such that the improved health of one improves the health of the other. A positive feedback loop is established with a healthier body improving the health of the mind, which then in turn improves the health of the body, and so on and so forth. We become in control of what was once out of our control. We become conscious of what is occurring in our bodies that was once hidden in the subconscious. A newfound connection develops between mind and body.

As yoga is considered a practice, as you arrive on your mat, through single-pointed focus to achieve mental clarity you are learning to relax. In a sense, you are practicing techniques to reorient your thinking away from habitual, automatic negative thoughts toward healthier perspectives and emotions. The hope is that what you learn through your practice of yoga will carry over to enjoy a full life experience.

Yoga becomes your sanctuary devoted to relaxation. Yoga brings you back to the safety of your cave where you can rest and take the time to focus on the positives in your life. It is a place of peace that you create, where all the blessings of life become visible.

As we practice yoga, we strive to maintain deep belly breaths, linking full inhalations and slow exhalations to the flow of movement. Although not fully understood, deep diaphragmatic breathing appears to activate the parasympathetic nervous system. Here lies one of the fundamental ways to consciously control the autonomic nervous system. Quite simply, deep breathing possesses the power to relax. Before moving on to the next chapter, perhaps take a few moments to close the eyes and focus on the sound of the breath as you inhale to complete fullness and exhale to complete emptiness. Sit back now and enjoy your power to relax!

5

A HEALTHIER BODY

Once we have realized the ability to bring the autonomic nervous system into a healthy balance with a reduction in the chronic stress of sympathetic overload and a newfound facility to access relaxed states, we can then begin to enjoy the positive benefits of our yoga practice on the physical health of the body. Your awareness of the improved health of the physical body can create positive feedback that can serve as further motivation to nurture the body by expanding your yoga practice. Feelings of pride become possible as you begin to face the once daunting challenges of overcoming the apparent uncontrollable negative influences of depression and anxiety. Improved physical health translates into improved mental health. The mind and body are not separate entities. Each has the power to influence the other. Ultimately, a dedication to self-care, including good nutrition, restorative sleep and, of course, yoga results in a healthier body.

This chapter explores the health benefits of a regular yoga practice, which can be best approached on the systems level. Systems are organs and tissues that act in concert to perform a particular function. The nervous system transmits information throughout the body. It is a bidirectional system in which electrical signals are sent to and from the brain. The cardiovascular system governs the delivery of blood and its essential components, including oxygen and nutrients, to the various organs and tissues of the body and the elimination of the byproducts of metabolism, including carbon dioxide and water. Gas exchange is the function of the respiratory system. Oxygen is inhaled and subsequently transferred into the blood, while unwanted carbon dioxide is extracted from the blood and subsequently exhaled. The immune system consists of the thymus gland, lymph nodes, specialized cells in the bone marrow and blood stream, and lymphatic channels that all work together to protect the body from disease. The musculoskeletal system is involved with movement. It is an intricate complex of bones that serve as the scaffolding for muscles, tendons, ligaments, fascia and joints that under the brain's direction move our bodies through space. The digestive system breaks down complex food into molecules that are small enough to be transported in the blood stream and enter into cells. It also eliminates anything ingested that the body can't use in the form of waste. The endocrine system governs the release of hormones in the brain and blood stream that have a multitude of functions, including the control of metabolism and the experience of mood.

Although the systems of the body have different functions, they all are interdependent on one another. For example, the cells of the nervous system, or neurons, require oxygen brought into the body by the respiratory system. That oxygen is transported to the neurons through the blood stream created by the pulsations of the heart and the presence of blood pressure. The neurons also require nutrients that are put in usable form by the actions of the digestive system and subsequently delivered by the cardiovascular system. Insulin, a hormone released from the pancreas, an endocrine organ, is delivered to the neurons by the cardiovascular system to stimulate the entry of the nutrient glucose into the cells. The immune system assures the health of the neurons. Finally, the neurons send impulses and signals to the organs and structures of all of the other systems, allowing the brain to direct this wonderful symphony that is the human body. Although these multiple systems of the physical body differ in function, all of the beneficial effects of yoga on their functioning and efficiency stem from the one source: the power of relaxation.

With regard to the cardiovascular system, a regular yoga practice builds endurance. During a yoga class, the heart rate typically increases, the magnitude of which is dependent on the vigor of the practice. Similar to other "cardio" exercises, over time the heart becomes stronger and more effective at delivering oxygen throughout the body, including to muscles and joints. With stronger and more effective contractions of the heart, the pulse rate drops, as less "beats" are required in a given time to deliver oxygen throughout the body. There is also a lessening of resistance to blood flow in the blood vessels reflected in a decrease in blood pressure. With decreased resistance to flow, the heart need not work as hard to generate the current of blood flow. Greater endurance can also translate into feelings of pride and accomplishment and a lessening of any negative self-judgments arising from perceived limitations to the full participation in many strenuous activities.

With regard to the respiratory system, the breath is central to the practice of yoga, both physically and spiritually. Listening and connecting to the breath promotes meditative states. From a physiological perspective, yogic breathing techniques, or *pranayama*, teach one how to optimize breathing capacity, thereby bringing more precious oxygen into the body that is necessary for the optimal functioning of all of the organs and muscles. Since the heart is also a muscle, more effective breathing also promotes greater cardiac efficiency. As mentioned previously, deep, diaphragmatic breathing has the power to trigger the parasympathetic nervous system, promoting states of physical and mental relaxation. Of course, diaphragmatic breathing need not be limited to one's yoga practice. It is the perfect tool to access during a busy and stressful day. Taking a moment to pause and take a deep breath that spreads from the belly to the upper chest like a gentle, relaxing wave can have the power to reset the mind and diffuse any distressing, uncomfortable thoughts, feelings and emotions.

Activating the parasympathetic nervous system through relaxation also has a beneficial effect on the digestive system. As discussed in the prior chapter, the parasympathetic system engages at times of safety and peace, allowing for a greater delivery of blood and oxygen to organs that are not vital in times of danger, including the stomach, small intestines and colon. Nourishing of these structures results in more effective digestion. Chronic anxiety overstimulates the sympathetic nervous system, reflected in poor bowel functioning and the so-called "pit in the stomach" feeling. Yoga allows one to rest and digest.

With regard to the immune system, a regular yoga practice can boost immunity and the body's defense mechanisms against disease. Chronic stress causes the release of cytokines and other circulating inflammatory molecules that can cause and worsen disease. The practice of yoga and learned relaxation can reverse that process, while, at the same time, alter the expression of genes involved in immunity.

With regard to the musculoskeletal system, yoga has widespread benefits that are realized in increased flexibility and strength and improved posture. Flexibility arises from the progressive stretching of muscle fibers, tendons, and ligaments. The stretching of the stiff connective tissues, or fascia that hold our joints together increases mobility and range of motion. Strength arises from the isometric effects of sustaining the postures. Although we are often unaware of it as we practice, almost all of the postures activate and engage the core. Strengthening the core, along with the conditioning of the spine, results in good posture, which can result in feelings of pride and confidence. One learns balance and grounding through yoga, both of which not only prevent falls, but also translates to a balanced, well-grounded life.

Finally, a regular yoga practice has widespread beneficial effects on the endocrine system. As mentioned, the endocrine system is involved in the secretion of hormones. Hormones are the body's chemical messengers. They are molecules that regulate the physiology of the body by delivering instructions to the various tissues and organs as how and when to function. They are relatively ubiquitous throughout our bodies, affecting the functioning and responses of the various systems, including the nervous, digestive, cardiopulmonary, and immune systems. They are commonly secreted by endocrine glands, travel to sites throughout the body and bind to receptors on cells in target organs and tissues. Here are just a few examples of the many hormones produced in the human body:

- *cortisol* and *epinephrine* - produced by the adrenal gland in times of stress
- *thyroxine* - produced by the thyroid gland to regulate metabolism

- *insulin* - produced by the pancreas to decrease blood and increase intracellular glucose
- *melatonin* - produced by the pineal gland in the brain to regulate sleep
- *gastrin* - produced in the stomach to increase gastric acid to aid in digestion
- *estradiol* - main female sex hormone produced in many organs, including the ovaries, which among other functions regulates the menstrual cycle
- *testosterone* - main male sex hormone produced in the testicles and to a lesser extent, the ovaries
- *parathyroid hormone* - produced by the parathyroid glands in the neck to regulate serum calcium levels

In the brain there are neurotransmitters that, like hormones, are chemical messengers but, unlike hormones, operate on a microscopic level between neurons. They are secreted by one neuron, or nerve cell, travel across the synapse, or space between neurons, and bind to receptors on an adjacent neuron. Four of the main neurotransmitters in the brain that impact mood are serotonin, dopamine, endorphins, and oxytocin, which to complicate matters, are also hormones, as they also function as chemical messengers that travel through the blood stream to more distant sites. I will now consider their roles, however, as neurotransmitters in the brain.

The term, "happy hormones" has been coined to refer to these four neurotransmitters. "Happy neurotransmitters" might be more accurate, but perhaps alliteration makes a name stick and more memorable. Physiologically, they have the potential to elicit feelings of happiness and pleasure, while reducing depression and anxiety. Factors relating to their release and re-uptake that affect their concentration in the synapses are numerous and quite complex, therefore I will attempt to simplify the long-term, beneficial effects of a regular yoga practice on levels of these neurotransmitters. It is important to stress the word "regular". Any activity or exercise will have a greater effect on the level of these molecules in the brain if done for longer periods of time and more frequently and regularly. An example is the "runner's high", which is reported more frequently in those that run often and for sustained periods of time. Such is true of yoga. Perhaps, it may be called a "yogi's high."

The four so-called "happy hormones" are:

Endorphins

Endorphin is a portmanteau created from the two words, endogenous and morphine. These are naturally occurring opiates, similar in structure to moprhine, that block the perception of pain, function as the body's natural painkillers, and can create feelings of wellbeing, and even euphoria.

Dopamine

Among the many functions of dopamine is its involvement in the brain's pleasure and reward system, helping to drive motivation and desire. Dopamine levels spike when you receive or anticipate receiving a reward.

Oxytocin

Oxytocin's primary function as a hormone is to stimulate contractions during labor and initiate lactation after birth. Its secretion is mediated by closeness and touch. In the brain, it is believed to bring about feelings of belonging, trust and intimacy, as well as modulate stress reactions. It is released during expressions of empathy and in meaningful and loving relationships.

Serotonin

Among its many roles throughout the body, including digestion, metabolism and sleep cycles, in the brain serotonin affects mood and can serve as an antidepressant. It can boost self-esteem and elicit feelings of wellbeing and contentment.

In summary:

- Endorphins are natural pain killers that can elicit feelings of wellbeing, and even euphoria
- Dopamine governs pleasure and reward
- Oxytocin elicits feelings of intimacy, belonging and trust
- Serotonin can boost self-esteem and elicit feelings of wellbeing and contentment

This, of course, is an extreme oversimplification. The actions and target sites for these "happy hormones" are too numerous to mention. The mechanism for their release is complex and multifactorial. Suffice it to say, however, regular activity, such as a yoga practice, can boost the levels of these chemical messengers, and therefore might be postulated to have an antidepressant effect. Many prescription antidepressant medications act to increase or decrease synaptic levels of some of these neurotransmitters. Along with other effects, bupropion, also known by the brand name Wellbutrin, boosts levels of dopamine. The class of antidepressants known as the SSRIs (selective serotonin re-uptake inhibitors), such as Prozac, Lexapro, Paxil and Zoloft, act to increase available serotonin levels in the synapse. It is entirely speculation, but might a regular yoga practice function as a dosing schedule of a natural antidepressant? As bears repeating, yoga is not a cure for mental illness, but a wonderful adjunct to and not a substitute for other therapies deemed necessary by your health providers. Once embraced, yoga becomes an effective coping mechanism and a path to mental wellness. One might even imagine that practicing yoga on a daily basis might function to create a steady state of increased levels of the "happy hormones", leading to a greater sense of self and wellbeing, promoting personal growth.

Many forms of exercise, including yoga, also decrease levels of monoamine oxidase and cortisol. Monoamine oxidase inhibitors (MAOI), such as Nardil and Parnate, have been used in the treatment of depression since the 1950's. Cortisol is a steroid, "stress" hormone that your adrenal glands produce and release. Cortisol has numerous functions, including helping to regulate your body's response to stress.

It is uncertain as to how a regular yoga practice leads to an increase in brain levels of the so-called "happy hormones". Whether it be activation of mechanoreceptors in fascia and muscles that initiate hormonal release, factors relating to changes in autonomic sympathetic-parasympathetic balance or conscious perceptions and expectations of peace and contentment, the practice of yoga can give us a literal emotional lift, as it causes the influx of "happy hormones" into the neural synapses of the brain.

Finally, I did not coin the term "happy hormones". When dealing with my mental illness, I don't strive to be happy. Rather, I wish for a lessening of psychic pain and mood swings, greater mental clarity and a semblance of peace of mind. I wish for a modicum of normalcy and a lessening of the mental static in order to appreciate the normal ups and downs of life. It might be a bad assumption, however, that normalcy exists at all, since all of us have our own genetics, personality development, past experiences, and perspectives that contribute to our different, unique thoughts and behaviors.

Through the aforementioned discussion, it is my hope that you have gained new perspectives concerning mood and the health of the physical body in the context of human physiology, thereby increasing the array of concepts available to you to consider while practicing your yoga. Once again, we strive to focus on what is occurring in the moment in order to divert thoughts away from rumination.

The science behind yoga supports the idea that a regular practice has widespread beneficial effects on our health and wellbeing. One must be so fortunate in life to be blessed with good health. Self-care increases your odds of enjoying that blessing. Take care of yourself. Your loved ones, friends and community depend on it. Embrace yourself and embrace life!

6

A HEALTHIER MIND

For years, my expectation was that I would suffer from depression and anxiety without end; that the mind was fixed. If this were the case, however, there would be no need to read this book or attempt anything novel to alter one's thinking and experiences in life for the better. I was not alone in my thinking. For decades, neuroscientists believed that once your brain matured, its structure was set in stone, like wet cement hardened into permanent grooves.

The precious ability to hope for the future lies in what is known as, "neuroplasticity"; literally the state of plastic nerves. Of course, plastic in this usage refers to something that is moldable. Rather than a fixed, unchangeable organ, the brain has been shown to be malleable, flexible, and dynamic. Like clay, it can be reshaped, especially with effort, attention, and repetition.

We witness neuroplasticity at work in stroke survivors who relearn how to walk or speak. Their brains, damaged in one area, often reroute tasks to other regions. And similarly through yoga, we can "rewire" the brain to bypass habitual reactions to stress in order to focus on the present moment and access states of calm and relaxation.

It is important to note that with neuroplasticity, changes that occur are not necessarily for the better. The brain can also rewire itself for fear, addiction, or anxiety if repeatedly exposed to trauma or stress. Neuroplasticity isn't inherently good or bad, but it can be a powerful force that can be harnessed for positive personal growth and transformation.

The power of yoga to transform exists in each and everyone of us. We just need to know how to access it. Like a huge boulder blocking the entrance to a cave, habitual and reflexive, negative thoughts and behaviors are obstacles that need to be moved in order to realize that power rather than remaining mired in emotional stagnation. The first step in reversing any trend is an awareness of the problem before an effective solution can be implemented. Learned relaxation through the practice of yoga promotes the mental clarity necessary for effective self-analysis. Negative thoughts are charged with emotions that cloud the mind. Mental clarity is achieved by becoming the objective witness of those thoughts, diffusing their emotional impact through observation and understanding.

Meditative states are achieved by deliberate single-pointed

focus. As mediative states deepen, an active mind relaxes and the magnitude of the emotional responses to disturbing thoughts and anxiety-laden negative self-judgements lessens. You then become positioned to analyze unhealthy thought processes that represent the problem and replace them with positive affirmations that represent the solution. This may seem like a lofty goal, which it is. For many of us who are works in progress, it may only be partially realized. Changing thought processes that are well established and ingrained into the psyche for years can require a herculean effort, but it is the work to be done to realize a degree of peace of mind. The technique of identification and analysis of automatic negative thoughts and the subsequent replacement of those thoughts with positive affirmations is at the heart of cognitive behavioral therapy, which has been shown to be very beneficial in the treatment of both depression and anxiety. A subset of the broader category of automatic, negative thought patterns is rumination on the chronic suffering inherent to depression and anxiety and concomitant feelings of hopelessness.

Changing thought patterns that have been ingrained for years may seem an insurmountable task, but making an attempt is better than doing nothing at all. Increasing your odds of success is prioritizing time for self-care. This is difficult for those that have busy lives, filled with obligations and responsibilities and a need for "veg out" time at the end of the day. It may seem like there is no way to carve out time for self-care. It seems paradoxical, but self-care activities like yoga reduce stress and heighten focus and concentration so they can actually create more time in your day by increasing productivity and efficiency. Their stress-reducing powers may also lessen the need to "stress eat" during "veg out" time at the end of the day, creating another opportunity to have control over what seems out of your control. Time set aside each day for yoga allows for mental clarity with a more consistent reinforcement of ideas and the opportunity for objective self-analysis of automatic negative thoughts and self-judgments that are typically falsely based in misinterpretations of reality. These unhealthy patterns of thought, or cognitive distortions, can cause or worsen anxiety and depression. Through self-reflection, we can analyze habitual ways of thinking and identify and categorize the particular cognitive distortions at play. The ability to distinguish between misperceptions and actualities must be developed before the process of substituting positive affirmations for negative self-judgments can begin.

An objective healthy inner dialogue is valuable before choosing how to emotionally react to a particular situation. A dependence on cognitive distortions, however, relieves the pressure to make that decision, leaving negative, self-deprecating feelings as the only option.

Taking a step back in order to examine all aspects of a stressful situation increases the probability of an appropriate, measured emotional response. In that regard, a practical technique known by the acronym BRFWA is taught at the Kripalu Center for Yoga and Health to both yoga instructors in training and participants in programs. BRFWA is an acronym that stands for *Breathe, Relax, Feel, Watch and Allow.* Many times during a busy day we become stressed or rushed or we become mired in thoughts that don't serve us, such as regrets of the past, worries about the future and rumination on the inability to control disturbing thoughts that stem from chronic depression and anxiety. Life can be a battle, but in your armamentarium, BRFWA can be a useful weapon.

- The first step is to notice the *Breath.* As we become stressed, breathing quickens and becomes more shallow. Focusing one's attention on deepening and slowing the breath is the first step to reestablish a calm state. Deep belly breathing triggers the parasympathetic response, activating the rest and digest system, unlike shallow chest breathing that results from greater sympathetic tone.

- The next step is *Relaxation.* Releasing and softening muscles while maintaining a deep breathing rhythm can dissipate feelings of stress. So many of us hold our tension in our muscles. Creating a focus on the breath and deliberately and consciously relaxing muscles diverts attention away from the stress-inducing thought or event.

- After establishing a deep breath and a relaxed, physical state, we notice how we *Feel.* What emotions or sensations can you become aware of?

Clarity of thought and recognition of specific emotions replaces an amorphous sense of how one is feeling.

- The next step, *Watch*, refers to observing your entire experience without attachment, that is, not embracing what is positive and pleasurable or avoiding that which is negative or distressing. It is an attempt to step out of oneself and become an objective witness to what has transpired. This is much easier said than done. One might imagine themselves as an umpire or referee that needs to look at the instant replay in order to settle a disputed call. The appropriateness of an emotional response to a stressful event can be better assessed by analyzing "the instant replay" in slow motion.

- Finally, you *Allow* by acknowledging the experience as it has unfolded, knowing that it was fine to react in your own way. This self-analysis can become habitual with practice. By understanding and embracing what has transpired, you can re-enter the present by letting go of the past. The end result is a revelation that you are enough as you are.

The main intention of BRFWA is simply an acceptance of yourself, your behaviors, your reactions and your emotions. In Western culture, there is a pervasive competitive attitude that too many of us possess, such that making mistakes becomes fraught with negative self-judgments. Perfection, however, is an unrealistic expectation. Recognizing that we all make mistakes promotes a healthier attitude of self-acceptance. Imagine how easy it would be to take care of your landscaping if we all loved the look of weeds and had no need to grow grass or manicure a lawn. We need not try to manicure our expressions and behaviors for the sake of appearances. Embrace yourself as you are, not how you think you need to be. Embrace your mistakes as opportunities for learning rather than resigning yourself to failure.

Another technique for self-realization that is taught at Kripalu is called, "Riding the Wave." The wave is composed of crescendoing anxiety and stress arising from a disturbing or distressing event. Before it crests, in order to escape the stress, many of us "jump" off of the wave, reverting to reflexive and automatic negative thoughts and behaviors, including negative self-judgments and well-established defense mechanisms. Learning more positive coping skills by having a full experience of a situation with greater understanding of its emotional impact is blocked. As a new wave of anxiety forms from another distressing event, one's response to stress remains unchanged. Each time one "jumps" off of the wave before it crests, opportunities for developing new perspectives and learning more positive attitudes are lost. Anxiety begets anxiety as a vicious cycle ensues. Remaining on the wave to experience its full emotional force is difficult. It requires tapping into one's inner strength to come face to face with painful and disturbing thoughts of feeling unsafe or out of control. Allowing the wave to crest, however, lets one appreciate the full impact of an experience, even if it is wrought with pain. As the wave begins to subside, we have an opportunity for self-analysis. Once the wave has fully abated and calm sets in, ensuing introspection might lessen future anxieties. Perhaps, what seemed unmanageable before now seems reasonable. Rather than being left to speculation, riding the wave can allow for a full understanding of the experience and our reactions to it. New healthier perspectives and greater resilience are now possible.

When I attended my first yoga class, a plethora of emotions and thoughts filled my head, mostly in the form of negative self-judgments. My feelings of low esteem inherent to my depression were exacerbated by thoughts of "not being good enough" or "others being able to do what I could not". I faced two choices. One option was to "jump off" the wave before it crested and succumb to my feelings of low self esteem inherent to my depression, never to move beyond my preconceived notions of yoga or return to another class. The other option, which I assure you I chose, was to push on and see what would unfold. That wave took quite a long time to crest. Anxiety persisted for weeks as I remained mired in false expectations and lamentations over my ineptitude in the many classes to follow. Once that wave crested, however, I was finally able to breathe. Through retrospective self-analysis, I came to identify and understand all of the factors that contributed to my anxiety as a novice in the world of yoga. With each class and online video, the waves of anxiety lessened in height and became more manageable over time. Even now, waves of self-doubt continue to crest as they roll into the shore, but they are smaller and more gentle than when I first began.

———

Often, facing the realities of life can be daunting, especially if one's past was difficult or traumatic. As a defense against the stress of taking on the truth with anticipated emotional discomfort we often distort reality. Cognitive distortions inherently are fraught with self-deprecation. They are in a sense short cuts; a detour around the unknowns of reality that, unfortunately, also bypasses the possibility of more positive, fulfilling experiences.

The following is a discussion of a few of the more common cognitive distortions. Deliberate labelling of a thought as a particular cognitive distortion can be a helpful exercise, although categorizing behaviors is not fully necessary to recognize unhealthy thought processes. Since this is a book about yoga, I will illustrate these cognitive distortions in that context. Eliminating cognitive distortions in our yoga practice can generalize to the other aspects of life, imbuing each day with a healthier outlook.

Comparison

Quite simply, self-criticisms arise from a comparison to others, which many do in yoga classes. Not very long ago, I was a novice at yoga. I made sure to get to the yoga studio early to get a spot for my mat in the back of the class so no one could watch me. Of course, I was under the misperception that everyone else knew what they were doing and could do all of the postures perfectly. I certainly couldn't. I had a defeatist attitude before I even began. As the class filled up, most people either sat or laid down on their mats and began to meditate. This made me feel even more uncomfortable and inadequate, as I had tried meditation in the past and absolutely hated it because of my inability to control all of the mind chatter. As class began, I concentrated on everyone in the room except myself. I neglected my own experience at the expense of an opportunity to assess whether or not my perceived limitations lay in reality. Of course, it was necessary for me to observe the teacher to understand the various postures and how to perform them. While I watched the teacher, however, my thoughts of my own inadequacy worsened. Here was this teacher who was so flexible that there seemed to be almost no position she couldn't assume. Faced with physical discomfort and an awareness of my inflexibility, I decided right then and there that there was no way that I would ever come close to performing the postures correctly. I was certain that I would be unsuccessful at yoga. At times, the teacher came over and corrected my position in a particular posture, seemingly more than other students in the class. Of course, it came as no surprise to me at the time that I was in the "wrong" position. Comparing myself to other people in the class magnified my negative self-judgments. I was so self-conscious. At the time, it seemed like they could all "do yoga" and I couldn't. They all knew the names of all of the postures. At times, the teacher even used the Sanskrit names for the *asanas* and it seemed that everyone else knew them except me. I spent an entire hour and fifteen minutes comparing myself to everyone, beating myself up for being what I perceived as being less than them. It is a miracle that I ever went back to a second class.

The cognitive distortion of comparison is not just particular to novices. Even many seasoned practitioners continue to do it, perhaps comparing their bodies or the performance of a posture to others. Our culture loves competition, from sports to reality television shows. We are compelled to compete with others and compete with ourselves, never dismissing a challenge because we can never just be satisfied with the way we are. Then, there is often that one person in a class who unsolicitously and spontaneously pops into an inversion posture, such as a headstand. My competitiveness would cause me to say to myself, "Showoff!" Comparison is a cognitive distortion that diverts attention away from one's self and towards others. By focusing on others' experiences, you miss out on your own.

Not infrequently, a yoga teacher will guide the class into a particular *asana*. He, she or they will then offer modifications. He, she or they might start you in a table position (on hands and knees) and instruct you to raise and extend one of your legs back at hip height. The teacher might then say something like, "You can stay here or if you want more of a challenge, you can raise and extend your opposite arm forward." "Then, for even more of a challenge, you can bend your knee and grab it with your raised hand." I have also heard teachers describe assuming a more strenuous variation of an *asana* as "adding more heat." Since, we are comparing ourselves to everyone else in what seems like this grand competition, we try to do whatever is the most extreme, difficult modification that the teacher suggests. I subscribed to this philosophy early on until I began to realize that some of these additional modifications were uncomfortable with the potential for injury.

When you go from a reasonably paced *Hatha* yoga class to a rigorous, fast-paced *vinyasa* flow or power yoga class, a comparison to others can result in even greater feelings of inadequacy. The pace of the postures can be so quick that there is little time to breathe between them. A failure to keep up can result in more negative self-judgments. Now, add some actual heat to the room so that everyone is sweating profusely and it might seem to you that yoga is a true competitive sport.

As the cognitive distortion of comparison becomes habitual, a lack of physical flexibility can allow the inner critic to squash any possibility for future success at yoga. When I first began, I was dismayed by the sight of fellow classmates sitting cross-legged with absolutely straight spines, while I sat with my knees high in the air with a rounded back and extreme discomfort in my inner thigh muscles. I beat myself up over my inability to sit properly. I was certain that yoga was not for me. I soon learned, however, that to properly sit cross-legged the knees should be below the level of the hips. This could be accomplished, or at least partially accomplished, by sitting on the edge of a bolster, which results in lifting the hips and dropping the knees. That insight allowed me to experience a small bit of progress. My knees were still up in the air, but now I could sit with a straighter spine. Unfortunately, my self-consciousness and competitive mindset got the better of me as I observed that no one else in the class was using a bolster. I felt that others must be watching me and that the bolster was a crutch and a visible sign of my inadequacy. Ultimately, more important than the insight into how to straighten my spine was the realization that the only person watching me that mattered was myself. Comparison to others in a yoga class clouds the mind and prevents gaining insight into our unhealthy thought processes.

Some talk about "yoga experiences": epiphanies and periods of clarity occurring during a yoga practice. As a beginner, I was skeptical of the existence of such "yoga experiences", but after several weeks of daily practice I began to develop some clarity as to how I wished to live each day. Although I remained somewhat mired in old habitual ways of thinking, I started to control the cacophony of negative thoughts in my head that prevented me from thinking about what was important in my life. I found myself more and more in the moment. I thought less about regrets of the past and worries about the future. With the lessening of the mind chatter, I could now enjoy my newfound ability to evaluate my life, including my desires, needs and goals. I realized that I no longer needed to be a version of myself that I thought others wanted me to be. I recognized my newfound control over how I wished to spend my day.

Although on many days, depression often gets the better of me, on others I can choose between a day filled with negativity or one full of positivity. When that happens, it is a very liberating experience that transfers the energy required to be negative to more productive pursuits. I accept that there will be days where I revert back to old habits that worsen my anxiety and depression, but my hope is that those days will occur less frequently. Most importantly, my yoga practice affords me a daily opportunity to acknowledge all of the blessings in my life. To this very day, it is gratitude that fills my heart. I pause during every class I teach or attend to experience that gratitude. I believe that gratitude is a prerequisite for all of the other positive emotions we experience. Your brain listens to everything you say. Positive affirmations become habitual after a while, replacing automatic and reflexive negative thoughts and behaviors.

With some of my self-judgments gone, my experience in classes has significantly changed for the better. My need to compare myself to others has lessened. I am not only less concerned about what others might think, but less aware of those around me. Often after a class, I can not tell you anything about any of my fellow students. Oblivious is not a good word. I prefer to think that I am in my own zone, a place of serenity I can now access.

Comparison to others is often unavoidable. Perhaps, it is part of human nature. Maybe one caveman felt compelled to see if another had a larger share of that day's hunt. In yoga as in life, arguably a much more healthy mindset is one of aware-ness and acceptance. Accepting limitations, either physical due to acquired or inherited inflexibility or mental due to acquired or inherited depression and anxiety, can free you from the constraints of unhealthy thoughts and emotions. Even more so, you might come to the realization that what you considered limitations are not limitations at all, that you are enough as the unique person you are. Focus on your abilities and talents and not on those of someone else.

Understanding the cognitive distortion of comparison in the context of a yoga class can generalize to other facets of daily life. By eliminating the need to compare, pride in your own talents can be felt, rather than shame from perceived limi-tations in the context of what someone else is doing. Rather than directing attention on the experience of others, direct it on yourself so that life doesn't pass you by.

Polarized Thinking

Also called black and white or all or nothing thinking,

polarized thinking is experiencing life in extremes. At its worst, small set-backs that others might consider small bumps in the road trigger feelings of complete failure. Despite successes in some aspects of yoga, polarized thinkers negate those successes and focus only on perceived failure. One might be enjoying their yoga practice until wobbling and falling out of a balance posture elicits lamentations about the possibility of never being able to do yoga. When I first began my practice, I would often find myself incapable of doing what the instructor was doing, which led me to dismiss any possibility of ever being able to practice yoga at all. I possessed an unhealthy mindset that caused me to ignore what I was capable of at the time. Layer that on my self-defeatist attitude from comparing myself to others, and I was doomed to fail.

The practice of self-observation without judgment can diminish polarized thinking. It is easier said than done, but leave out the word "and" from your thoughts. Instead of thinking, "I am wobbling and I will never be good at balance postures", simply observe, "I am wobbling." The second part of the sentence doesn't serve you. By not judging yourself as either good or bad, there is an opportunity to exist somewhere between all or nothing. In yoga, having it all is an unrealistic expectation and having nothing is a false belief that is not based in reality.

In the practice of yoga, polarized thinking is also diminished through non-attachment to the possibilities of success or failure. It is being fine with whatever outcome might result. By not being preoccupied with the end result, you can better focus on the present moment and enjoy the process. Entering into a balance posture without concern for whether or not you will be able to stand on one leg expands the mental space available for single-pointed concentration on your *drishti*. In essence, a balance posture is not a physical challenge, but rather a mental one. True success at the pose is not defined as being able to stand on one leg, but rather achieving single-pointed focus. Arguably, the person that keeps both feet on the ground, but is able to maintain a focus on a *drishti* is more successful than one who wobbles on one leg; their mind filled with thoughts of wobbling and potential negative self-judgments arising from an inability to physically balance.

Like the cognitive distortion of comparison, an understanding of your use of polarized thinking in your yoga practice can carry over into other aspects of life. Non-attachment to success or failure can become a generalized sense that you are more than fine as you are.

Mind Reading

Mind reading is a cognitive distortion whereby one assumes they know what someone else is thinking. It stems from a complete lack of communication. If I ask someone to express their thoughts, their intentions are no longer up to speculation. If I bump into an acquaintance and they seem cold and distant, mind reading may take the form of statements like, "They don't like me" or They're not interested in what I have to say." If I had an opportunity to ask how my acquaintance was feeling, I might find that he, she or they is depressed, having a bad day or grieving; their detached attitude having nothing to do with me. Feelings of low self-esteem and a lack of opportunity for open communication are inherent to mind reading. It is a cognitive distortion that involves replacing negative self-judgments for accurate information. When I was a novice in a yoga class, my own self-consciousness turned into a belief that everyone else thought I was inept. The likely truth was that no one was that interested in me. I also disregarded the possibility that others in the class might be supportive and kind. I simply did not know. I once again took a short cut to thoughts that reinforced my own negative judgments rather than having to face the stress stemming from facing the unknown that exists in reality.

Like all cognitive distortions, mind reading is a misinterpretation of reality that can become habitual. Through yoga, we can learn to quiet the mind by being mindful of the moment in a quest for self-satisfaction; being content with who we really are; focusing on what we are thinking and not what others might be.

Shoulda, Coulda, Woulda

"What's past is prologue" is a quote from *The Tempest* by William Shakespeare. Past experiences form the context for expectations for our interactions that occur in the present. A deliberate, conscious choice can be made between focusing on perceived failures with "shoulda, coulda, woulda" statements versus realizing that an analysis of past experiences represents a learning experience to increase the odds for success in the future. Of course, ultimately non-attachment to future outcomes should be our guiding principle, which increases the more important odds of being in the moment and enjoying the process; relieving the need to perform. A realistic exploration of prior life experiences creates a potential for learning better ways to cope in the present.

Catastrophizing

Catastrophizing is considering the worst possible outcome no matter how improbable it might be. Many times, this cognitive distortion manifest as "what if" questions. "What if she didn't answer her phone because she got into an accident?" Of course, that is in the realm of possibility, but there are many other more likely reasons for not answering a phone. Perhaps, the phone ran out of charge, there is no cellular service, or she is on another call, to name just a few.

"What if he didn't show up for lunch because I said something he didn't like?" Once again, that is in the realm of possibility, but by stepping back from that thought, other plausible possibilities become apparent. Possibly, he got caught in traffic, his meeting ran late or he entered the wrong time into his calendar, again to name just a few alternative explanations.

Superstitiousness is a close relative of catastrophizing. There is a compulsion to consider the most disastrous outcome in order to prevent it from happening. If I worry about the plane crashing it certainly won't happen. This is a self-reinforcing pattern of thought since probabilities are in favor of less extreme outcomes. The percentage of commercial flights that crash is relatively infinitesimal, but since it didn't crash, I can falsely conclude that my superstitious thinking worked. In all likelihood the worst possible scenario will not occur, which reinforces the belief that it was prevented by considering it in the first place. Superstitiousness is a type of magical thinking not based in reality that is an unreasonable attempt to control that which is out of one's control.

Filtering

Filtering is distilling out all positive aspects of a situation and fixating solely on the negative. For example, due to my inability to assume the full expression of a particular *asana*, I negate all of the other enjoyable aspects of my yoga practice. The brain listens to what you say. If you only tell it about your deficiencies, it will never come to know and enjoy your abilities. As a novice, I would focus on the pain and discomfort I experienced in some of the poses, while discounting the many aspects of yoga I enjoyed. It took quite a while to focus on what

I could do in order to enjoy my experience. An unrealistic expectation is that everything in yoga feels good. There may be poses or ideas that are uncomfortable. Recognize them and modify your practice and thinking to honor both body and mind. In life, it is also an unrealistic expectation to expect that everything will be pleasing. It is unavoidable that there will be many aspects of life that make you uncomfortable, both emotionally and physically. Don't filter out the joy in life by fixating on those disturbing thoughts. Rather, recognize them and modify your daily experience to minimize discomfort and stress.

Generalization

Generalization is when a setback or perceived failure carries over into more global thinking. "I can't balance and I am terrible at everything I try!" Generalization is especially troublesome in the setting of mental disease since inherent to clinical depression are general feelings of low self-esteem, which are magnified and reinforced by any perceived failure. A healthier way to think is to not generalize, but be more specific regarding your experience of what you are attempting in the present moment, whether it be an *asana* or a task at work, and once again practicing non-attachment to possibilities or success or failure.

Magnification

Magnification is ascribing greater significance to a perceived failure disproportionate to its actual importance. I try to ask myself when I lament my inability to assume a particular pose, "Just really how important is this in the grand scheme of my life?" Moreover, a failure may not necessarily be perceived accurately. In yoga, true failure arises from lamentations and negative self-judgments at the expense of enjoying and relaxing into your experience. Perhaps, rather than magnifying the importance of failure, emphasize your successes with pride.

Cognitive distortions are defense mechanisms. Unfortunately, they offer protection from dangers that are unfounded in reality. Our proverbial caveman would live an unhealthy existence filled with chronic anxiety if he always feared a saber-toothed tiger attack every time he left the cave. His spear would always be ready in hand, but his arm would fatigue. Similarly, habitually distorting reality leads to a fatigue of the mind. Cognitive distortions are charged with the emotional power to slowly erode the spirit. Habitual, automatic negative thoughts and behaviors induce chronic stress states that insidiously cause a decline in general health and a greater susceptibility to disease.

Once we establish mental clarity through learned relaxation, we are better equipped to develop a healthier way of thinking. This requires three main steps. The first requires gaining an awareness of cognitive distortions, possibly categorizing them as one of the aforementioned types. The second step involves dispelling the myth propagated by the cognitive distortion. The third, and possibly the most difficult step, is the substitution of positive affirmations for negative, self-deprecating thoughts.

I will illustrate this three-step process by using myself as an example. I began my practice of yoga five years ago. At that time, I carried tension in my muscles that developed over many years. I was physically inflexible. I was unable to sit cross-legged or touch my toes. I had tried yoga sporadically over the years, but never for long, not only because of physical discomfort and pain, but also due to my unhealthy, habitual thought patterns. I compared myself to others in the class, convinced I would never be able to do what they could do. I was guilty of mind reading. I was convinced everyone was watching me and noticed my ineptitude. I filtered out anything that was pleasurable from my experience. I was guilty of polarized thinking. Fixating on my physical and mental discomfort led me to the conclusion that I would never be good at yoga. Through the cognitive distortion of generalization, that conclusion reinforced the idea that I wasn't that great at anything I tried. Like many things in my life, I "shoulda" never have tried it. As you can see, cognitive distortions are usually not isolated ways of thinking, but more often become layered, one on top of the other, worsening their impact more so than if each one was employed separately. This is analogous to an exposure to a loud piercing siren. Now, layer on a cacophony of sounds emanating from the members of a marching band all playing different music and the result will likely be unbearable. Through deliberate self-analysis, I accomplished the first step and identified and categorized those cognitive distortions on which I relied.

With regard to the second step, I am still a work in progress, and likely will always be one, but after gaining some awareness of my distorted thinking, I can reflect on the reality of my situation. I can dispel the myths of my distorted thinking. To do so, I posed many questions to myself. How important was it that I could or couldn't do whatever everyone else was doing? Did I truly believe that everyone knew exactly what they were doing and were physically capable of doing everything? I wasn't judging anyone else, so why did I think others would be judging me? The reality was that many in the class were not capable of the full expression of all of the *asanas*. I wasn't thinking that they were any less deserving of respect and kindness, so why should I feel that they didn't respect me or weren't kind? Once I realized that the only right way to do yoga was to make it my own personal experience of the connection of my breath to my own unique movements, I no longer let my physical limitations negate the possibility of an enjoyable yoga practice. I recognized that my expectation that every posture was comfortable and accessible to me was an unrealistic one. Consequently, I stop filtering to allow for the full experience of my practice with a consideration of both what I could do and couldn't. I diminished the importance of perceived failures to better enjoy the moment, focusing on more positive and productive thoughts. If I found myself in a yoga class that was too vigorous and fast-paced I dropped the "shoulda" or "coulda" done something differently type of thinking. Rather, I chose to modify my experience to honor my body and lessen any risk of injury. Typically, if my body tires, child's pose is my go to, dismissing the misconceived notion that anyone is judging me because I took a body break.

The final step remains the most difficult one for me. Substituting positive affirmations for my reflexive negative self-judgments means I must like myself. This is a difficult task for one that has suffered with the self-loathing of depression for years. There are still times that I don't like myself much, but through my yoga I have newfound pride in my abilities and body. I have learned to practice self-kindness, love and compassion. That has enabled me to have more love and compassion for others. I learned that by comparing myself to others, I was missing out on observing my own experience. Instead of worrying about what others thought of me, I could give myself credit for taking care of myself regardless of my abilities. I began to focus on what I could do, and not what I couldn't. I finally learned what it means to "do" yoga and realized I was capable of doing it from the very start. I have a long way to go, but I am proud of the progress I have made in being

---

able to affirm my good qualities and accomplishments. At times, I find I can breathe deeply into words of self-love: I am capable, I am proud, I am grateful.

The brain listens to everything it hears. At first you may not believe that you are worthy, capable or deserving of love, but if you begin to affirm your self-worth, after a while you might find yourself believing it, even at least just a little. That tiny new belief can become a seed. Noticing that a positive outlook simply feels good may make you desire more. Often, repeating something over and over causes it to morph into a true belief. A laugh yoga class in which I participated is a perfect example. At the beginning of class, the teacher told us that even if we didn't find anything funny, just fake laughing anyway. With an inability to emotionally let go, I assumed I would be pretending to laugh for the entire class. My brain, however, was hearing my laughter and the laughter of others and, to my surprise, after a short time I was uncontrollably, hysterically laughing. Sometimes, you just have to let go. Letting go of ingrained, unhealthy thought patterns can lessen stress and ameliorate the symptoms of depression and anxiety. Yoga is a practice of release; letting go of physical tension and thoughts that press down on the spirit.

As you practice yoga, entering into stillness represents the best opportunity to connect with yourself. Resting the mind and body facilitates self-analysis, an understanding of reflexive, negative thoughts that are based in a distorted reality and an affirmation of your self-worth. A realistic expectation is that a transition from negative thinking to healthier perspectives takes time. You may never fully detach from ingrained defense mechanisms, but ultimately there is a realization that you can choose how and what to think. Mental disease tries to convince you otherwise, but you possess the power to choose self-kindness over self-hatred and self-worth over self-loathing. You can consider life situations from many different perspectives. Learned relaxation lets you choose the perspective, which at the very least doesn't make you feel uncomfortable. The perspective you choose, however, has the potential for a new positive outlook on life and a healthier mind.

As previously mentioned, learned relaxation through yoga creates a sanctuary. One might imagine stepping into a beautiful space that you design, possibly with bright sunshine passing through sparkling stained glass, projecting colorful patterns on the floor, or a fountain producing the peaceful sounds of bubbling water. However you envision your sanctuary, it is a safe place where nothing "bad" is happening at the present moment. Your inner critic isn't allowed to enter your sanctuary. In your safe space, there is no need and no pressure for criticisms and self-deprecation. Its peace is your peace. Its inner beauty is your inner beauty. It is a dedication to yoga that will provide you with the key to unlock the door that opens into your place of safety, beauty and peace.

7

THE EXTERNAL WORLD AND THE INTERNAL SELF

As we practice yoga, we strive to heighten our awareness of the experience in order to clear the mind of thoughts that don't serve us in the present. In a Hatha yoga class, the majority of the time is devoted to strengthening, stretching and experiencing all that is happening in the physical body. This, in part, is due to the relative loss of time spent in *pranayama,* or the yogic breathing techniques, in the Western world, but also secondary to the physical nature of the tradition and philosophy of Hatha yoga. In that regard, *Hatha* is a Sanskrit word that means "force". Much of what we know of Hatha yoga comes from the *Hatha Yoga Pradipika,* a seminal book written in the 15th century by Svatmarama and based on the teachings of the 11th century great sage Matsyendranath. He introduced a physical practice that could serve as a vehicle to obtain spirituality. Masters of Hatha yoga also advanced the idea of a life force or *prana* that activates the subtle body. *Prana* is received into the body with the breath, and then flows to the deeper self and spirit. Once *prana* is brought in from the external world, it then must be balanced throughout the body. To that end, a system of energy centers, or *chakras,* and channels, or *nadis,* was proposed that facilitate the flow of *prana.* Thus, they believed in an intimate interaction of the external world with the internal self.

From a historical perspective, I believe that what the ancient yogis professed was an early attempt to describe human anatomy and physiology. Perhaps, *prana* is what we now know as oxygen, which supports our life force. Analagous to the proposed thousands of *nadis* are trillions of nerve cells that transmit information throughout our bodies, including to the brain where we can consciously appreciate what our body is telling us at any given moment in time.

We are all familiar with the fives senses: touch, smell, taste, hearing and sight. The five senses each represent an intricate and extensive complex of receptors and neural networks that allow us to experience and appreciate the external world around us within the internal self. The sensation of the touch of a foot on your yoga mat is an experience of something in the external world, as is true of a smell, a sound, an visual image, or a taste. The five senses collect information from the external world and constantly update us as to what is occurring around us. Focusing on that information with a clear mind is at the core of the practice of mindfulness.

Along with the five senses that let us know what is happening in the external world, there exists "internal" senses that relay signals to the brain, furnishing it with information about what is occurring within the physical body. These internal senses include pain, stretch, and proprioception, or the sense of where the body exists in space. These three internal senses provide further information to the brain, providing additional sources for practicing mindfulness.

Finally, the sense that lacks a definable scientific basis is insight. In yogic philosophy, the *ajna chakra* or third eye governs the energy devoted to insight. Unlike our two eyes that only see the external world, the third eye can peer inward. If developed and carefully nurtured over time, this sense allows us to see deeply within to discover our true relationship of the external world with the internal self. It allows us to assess our true authenticity as we interact with the world around us, including the way we emotionally connect and react to cultural and societal norms and external and self-imposed expectations.

I will first consider the practice of mindfulness and the experience of the five senses, then the act of listening to the three internal senses of the physical body, and, lastly, the sense of insight, which lies at the heart of learned relaxation and coping with whatever mental challenges you face.

Mindfulness literally means "the state of a full mind". I believe, however, that it is just the opposite; an empty mind focused only on a single thought. Immersion into a single idea gives you the power to eliminate thoughts that don't serve you and lessens the stress that presses down upon the spirit. Once again, learned relaxation is realized through single-pointed focus on whatever is occurring in the present moment.

There are many wonderful books written about mindfulness. I especially recommend the writings of Thich Nhat Hanh, a Buddhist monk, teacher and political activist who many consider the father of mindfulness. In the following discussion, I will focus on mindfulness as a tool to elicit feelings of inwardness and introversion through a heightened awareness of physical sensations that are experienced on your yoga mat, promoting mindfulness and triggering thoughts and ideas that are manifestations of your interpretation of the external world. Yoga affords us the opportunity to exercise personal choice. The single object on which you focus should be one that piques interest and stimulates the mind.

Achieving single-pointed focus depends on clearing the mind of other thoughts, which is facilitated by the realization that one is safe on their mat and nothing bad is happening at that moment. Once we feel safe and in control, we can relax. With depression and anxiety, things often just seem out of control. The practice of mindfulness through yoga may not fully eliminate those feelings, but a revelation can occur that there is something that is in your control; quite simply, choosing where to focus your attention.

A classic mindfulness exercise to employ all of the five senses uses a Hershey's Kiss:

- *Vision* ~ one can explore the appearance of the Kiss; the glint of light reflecting off of the silver, metallic, wrinkled foil wrapper and the wispy, white paper ribbon sticking out the top.
- *Hearing* ~ one can experience the sound of a finger running over the wrapper.
- *Smell* ~ once the Kiss is unwrapped, the sweet scent of milk chocolate can be experienced.
- *Touch* ~ the tactile experience of the Kiss changes as it is unwrapped. Once placed in the mouth, the touch sensations experienced on the tongue continually change as the Kiss melts. Once the Kiss is almost liquefied, the feel of the teeth pushing into the soft chocolate can be appreciated.
- *Taste* ~ the evolution of the taste is appreciated as the chocolate slowly melts. The melting chocolate continues to stimulate the sense of smell receptors because of the continuity of the nasopharynx and oropharynx, the physical connection of the nose and mouth. Swallowing the Kiss creates a taste sensation on the back of the throat where additional taste buds exist.

The doorway to a state free from anxiety and stress opens into mindfulness-based yoga. Through yoga, by using all of our senses, we create a string of thoughts that keeps us in the moment for a protracted period of time. The object of one's focus is an individual choice. Personalizing your practice is part of "doing" yoga. Once again, the only right way to do yoga is to make it your own experience that speaks to you, and you alone, reflecting the unique person that you are. Your object of focus can also vary from moment to moment. The scope of self-observation can widen by employing all of the senses.

To apply mindfulness to the practice of yoga, we simply need to ask how each of the five senses can be experienced. Since we wish to generate one thought at a time by employing one sense at a time, eliminating as many of the other senses as possible facilitates single-pointed concentration. You likely would be better able to observe the tonal qualities of a particular sound if a strong odor was eliminated, and vice versa. I could be more aware of the touch of my palms on my yoga mat if I wasn't simultaneously stimulating my sense of taste with a Hershey's Kiss in my mouth.

Arguably, most effective in facilitating single-pointed focus is eliminating visual stimuli while engaging the other senses. Millions of bits of data flood our constantly moving eyes each second, converting light into electrical signals that course throughout the brain. Attempting to focus on a physical sensation other than a visual one with the eyes open is analogous to trying to find a needle in a haystack. Eliminating visual stimuli is like removing all of the hay; the needle being a sound, scent, taste, touch, or one of the three internal senses. Closing the eyes removes visual data, allowing the brain to better process signals arising from the other senses. Therefore, if physical balance is not my goal and imbalance is not an issue for the particular *asana* I am sustaining, I prefer to close my eyes while practicing yoga.

Of course, it is important to recognize that in a yoga class not everyone is comfortable closing the eyes in a room full of people. Just as one should not overstretch a muscle due to physical pain, one should not do anything in yoga that results in mental discomfort.

Although the brain processes a magnitude greater amount of visual data, bombarding any of the senses with unwanted information is antithetical to the goal of achieving single-pointed focus. For example, with regard to the sense of hearing, if I were riding in a crowded subway car filled with a marching band playing random notes while alarm bells ring, I would have extreme difficulty focusing on the sound of my breath. An environment that, in a sense, simplifies our sensual experience is more effective at promoting single-pointed focus than one filled with heavy "mental traffic."

Whatever your point of focus becomes, it is paramount that it is what demands your attention. Filling your mind with a single thought may seem an unachievable ideal. Yoga is a practice, however, and we are all works in progress. You might even consider that discovering that your mind has been distracted or wandering can actually be beneficial, as it represents an awareness of what your mind is doing at the moment, allowing you to acknowledge thoughts as they arise and return back to your object of single-pointed focus.

Opportunities also arise to redirect your concentration to different points of focus, such as successively changing your awareness of different points of touch, possibly shifting from the sensation of the touch of the palm on the mat to the feeling of the foot. Possibly, you might shift from the use of one sense to another, such as first noticing a point of contact on your mat and then listening to the sound of your breath.

In the following exploration of mindfulness, it is best to discuss each of the senses in the context of yoga separately. Again, you always possess the freedom to shift attention from one sense to another at any time during your practice. My sincere desire is to give you a clear "sense" of what it means to be mindful.

Vision

Visualizing a single point with unwavering focus is tricky. Our eyes are constantly darting in all directions. We must steady the gaze to establish a single point of focus. In yoga, we call this a *drishti, a* Sanskrit word that translates to "focused gaze". We don't wish to just simply stare at a single point, however. Rather, deliberate observation and examination of all of the qualities and characteristics of your *drishti* is much more effective at creating mental clarity. For example, if my *drishti* is a leaf on a tree, I can observe its shape, color or patterns, adding to the richness of my experience. My observations draw all thought to the qualities of the leaf. And at the risk of sounding cliche, I might even experience a "oneness" with the leaf.

We often speak of establishing a *drishti* before entering into balance postures since it facilitates physical balance. Observing a single point diverts thinking away from the state of the physical body. Often in a balance posture, negative self-judgments arise from wobbling or falling out of a pose. One might even enter into the pose with a self-fulfilling prophecy that physical balance is not possible. It is important not to give too much importance to the ability to stand on one leg, but rather adopt a healthier attitude that additional attempts to achieve physical balance come at no additional cost. Removing the pressure to perform frees up more mental space for detailed observation of your *drishti*.

When choosing a *drishti* in a class, I prefer one on the floor. You are less aware of and distracted by other people's movements. In addition, the *drishti* is more impactful when connected to the breath. When we attempt to balance, we often hold our breath and tense the body. Deep, diaphragmatic breathing relaxes the body, and when directed at our *drishti* intensifies its presence. One might imagine the *drishti* being drawn closer and closer to the eyes with each deep inhalation.

Paradoxically, physical balance might be achieved with the eyes closed by employing a technique known as "internal gazing." As was mentioned, the eyes are constantly darting back and forth, including when the eyes are closed. By directing the eyes to the third eye center, the eyes can become motionless. A single point that represents the third eye can be imagined serving as your "internal" *drishti*.

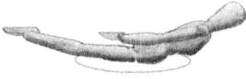

Salabhasana ~ the Grasshopper

Observation of a *drishti* is not exclusive to balance postures. For example, in *salabhasana*, the grasshopper pose, in which one is supine with chest, arms and legs all lifted from the mat, one might establish a *drishti* on the front edge of the mat. Heightened concentration on that point can divert attention away from the physicality of this demanding, vigorous pose, possibly allowing one to sustain it for longer periods of time. Layering on deep diaphragmatic breathing causes the body to gently rise and fall with each inhalation and exhalation while maintaining an unwavering gaze upon your *drishti*.

Hearing

Yoga is a breath-oriented practice. With the sense of hearing, we can appreciate the tonal quality of the breath as it flows in and out of the nose. As the breath deepens, the sound evolves into the peaceful sounds of ocean waves. Increasing the volume of the sound with *ujjayi* breathing, which I will discuss in more detail in a subsequent chapter, fills the mind with a sense of serenity.

Many other opportunities exist for being mindful of sounds. The use of music in a yoga class or personal practice can promote meditative states. The emotional content of music runs the gamut from joy to solemnity. Music that explores the intimate interrelationship and tonal qualities of sound, such as the sweet sounds of Buddhist prayer bowls, can be a wonderful object of your focus.

In many Eastern religions, meditative states are achieved through the repetition of mantras. Mantras can also be sung to music, producing a vibratory energy with frequencies that promote a calm mind. One example of a chanted mantra is *"Ra Ma Da Sa Sa Say So Hung"*, a Kundalini yogic mantra for healing that activates all of the *chakras*. Each of the seven words chanted represent each of the *chakras*. The words have an alternate translation, as well:

- *Ra* means the sun, and chanting it allows one to harness its energy.
- *Ma* is the moon, which is calming and cool, allowing one to become more receptive to new ideas and perspectives.
- *Da* is the earth, which elicits feelings of safety.
- *Sa* and *say* represent different aspects of the infinite.
- *Hung* means "I am thou".

The chanting of a single mantra for a relatively long time maximizes its meditative effects. In yoga, when set to music, those meditative effects can be better realized by connecting the pace of physical movements to the tempo of the music.

Touch

As you are reading this book, take a moment and scan the body, observing what each part of the body is touching or what is touching it. You may sense the feel of your feet on the ground or maybe the sensation of your socks wrapping the feet and toes. You might notice the touch of your pants on your legs or your shirt on your chest and arms. Take your time and focus on one point of the body at a time. Mindfulness using the sensation of touch is a powerful tool to achieve a single point of focus that exists in the present moment. A similar exercise can be performed on the yoga mat where awareness can evolve into observation and analysis. A knee resting on the mat elicits a thought initiated by receptors in the skin that send signals to the brain. The focus on the knee might evolve into an examination of portions of the knee that seem to take on more weight than others or an awareness of the touch of pants or leggings interposed between skin and mat. Greater awareness is achieved by coupling the breath to these sensations. Return to the above exercise. This time as you scan your body, breathe deeply into the awareness of each point and notice an intensification of the physical sensations.

Taste

The sense of taste is arguably the least accessible of the five while on a yoga mat. We might, however, imagine instances where taste might come into play. Perhaps, one might taste the saltiness of perspiration on the face in a vigorous practice. Possibly, one can enjoy a tasty drink to hydrate during a break. And as we strive to practice yoga on and off of the mat, we can nurture ourselves and promote wellbeing through mindful eating. As in our Hershey Kiss exercise, each sense is better appreciated when experienced alone. In that regard, you might try an experiment. The next time you eat something, tap your finger on the table. Bring all of your concentration to the sound of the tapping finger as you chew and swallow. For your next bite, moving only your jaw to chew, focus solely on the sensation of taste. Notice the greater appreciation of flavor when your attention is directed solely on the evolution of tastes in your mouth. Mindful eating includes slowing down and chewing more. Digestion begins in the mouth. Chewing breaks food into smaller pieces, thereby increasing surface area and the consequent greater effectiveness of digestive enzymes in the upper gastrointestinal tract. Chewing longer allows more time for amylase and lipase in saliva to digest starches and fats, respectively. Of course, the longer you chew, the more time you have to savor your food. So take your time and enjoy one of the true sensual pleasures in life.

Smell

Similar to taste, one is usually not mindful of odors during a yoga practice. Of course, hopefully body odor is not an issue, which is certainly a distraction from any attempt to focus.

Much more conducive to being attentive is mindfulness of a pleasant scent, possibly emanating from a candle or oils dispersed into the air from a diffuser. Once again, the goal is the awareness of the scent without any other physical sensation or thought. Conscious and deliberate suppression of thoughts in order to concentrate on one thing at a time is part of learned relaxation, the ability of which ultimately fades into the subconscious mind with time.

Although we most often consider mindfulness in the context of the five senses, in our yoga practice we can also be mindful of the three internal senses: proprioception, stretch and pain.

Proprioception

Proprioception is an awareness of the position of the body in space. Proprioceptors are organelles that are ubiquitous throughout the muscles, tendons and joints of the muscu-loskeletal system that react to and send signals to the brain about changes in body position. They possess complex mechanisms to sense the forces of gravity on the body as it moves. To experience proprioception, close your eyes, then raise your right arm out at shoulder height and then above your head. Although you weren't visualizing your arm, through your sense of proprioception you know exactly where it is in space.

Repeat the same motion, but when your hand comes overhead, bend your index finger. Notice how all your focus and
attention are directed solely to the movement and changing
position of your finger. You were probably not thinking about
anything else for that moment, including the past or the
future. You were mindful of the movement of your finger and
your mind was filled with a single thought, even if it was only
for a fleeting moment. As you can see, we can practice mindfulness by engaging the five senses, but also by focusing on
one of the internal ones.

The sense of proprioception is often overlooked, but is
central to the experience of mindfulness through the practice
of yoga. The body assumes a position specific to each *asana*.
Despite the accepted ideal full expression of a yoga pose, each
one of us has unique ways of positioning the body such that no
one assumes a specific *asana* like anyone else. While in a pose,
through proprioception, the brain knows where each body
part exists in space.

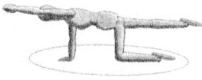

Chakravakasana ~ The Sunbird

As it bears repeating, that awareness
is enhanced by eliminating the flood of
visual data by closing the eyes if possible. Similar to the use of the sense of
touch, scanning the body is an effective
method to experience proprioception
one point at a time. Consider the *asana, chakravakasana,* the
sunbird pose. While scanning the body, one could notice the
position of the outstretched arm in space. With eyes closed,

one knows exactly where the arm is positioned. One might shift focus to the position of the outstretched leg or the chest, pelvis or neck. Once again, breathing into the awareness of a particular sense intensifies the sensation, in this case the position of each body part.

Stretch

One of the many pleasures of life is a good, full body stretch, especially upon awakening. Stretch receptors are a type of mechanoreceptor that respond to the stretching or deformation of the tissue in which they are embedded. These can be found in the airways of the lungs regulating inflation and deflation of the lungs, especially regulating overinflation to prevent pulmonary injury. They are also found in blood vessels, sensing stretch in the smooth muscle of arteries to help regulate blood pressure. As we practice yoga through mindfulness, we are most interested in the stretch receptors present in the muscles, tendons, joints and fascia. As we stretch a muscle, the stretch receptors convert mechanical into electrical energy in the form of neural impulses. The electrical signal in the neurons is transmitted to and subsequently up the spinal cord, delivering information to the brain. With our "good stretch", a part of that information is delivered to the pleasure centers of the brain with the release of some of the "happy hormones", discussed in the prior chapter. A yoga practice provides a constant opportunity to experience pleasure through stretching, which is more than welcome for those of us who suffer through the pain of depression and anxiety. By focusing on the internal sense of stretch, we can bombard the brain with pleasurable sensations, which over time can replace some of the mental real estate devoted to the pain and discomfort of mental illness. Of course, we wish to prevent discomfort through overstretching by practicing on our edge, so that the information provided to the brain is not diverted away from our pleasure centers, which brings us to our third internal sense, that of pain.

Pain

An important part of our nervous system and ubiquitous throughout the body are millions of pain receptors, or nociceptors, that detect potential harm to the physical body. One might postulate that these developed evolutionarily to promote survival by guarding against potential mortal injury. As we practice, we might think of nociceptors as millions of tiny alarm bells that are set off by the overstretching of muscles, tendons and fascia or undue stress on joints. The alarm bells might signify that injury has occurred, but pain can also alert one to possible impending injury. The latter scenario allows us to react with adjustments that bring us back to a safer place physically. It is paramount to always listen for these alarm bells and modify your practice to eliminate discomfort, which often can precede pain and be a harbinger of potential injury. Although we wish to be mindful of the internal sense of pain, it cannot coexist with pleasure or relaxation. In that regard, listen to your body and modify your practice in order to turn your attention back to any of the other senses that we can experience and enjoy.

Insight

This sense is the function of the third eye or *ajna chakra*, the energy center for awareness that is located in the center of the forehead. Unlike our two other eyes that can only see the external world, the third eye allows us to see inward with insight, with the power to elicit emotions and thoughts that connect mind and body and, ultimately, a connection to one's true self. The third eye also allows us to appreciate the emotional impact of our observations that are made with our other two eyes.

One ascends through six *chakras* before fueling the energy of the seventh *sahasrara chakra* at the crown of head, the energy center for spirituality. The sixth position of the third eye *chakra* just below the crown of head implies that self-knowledge and wisdom are the final steps necessary to connect to one's spirit. The sense of insight lets us peer into and possibly create an intimate connection to the inner self. Becoming the objective observer leaves one in a better position to analyze thoughts and emotions in a productive manner. Similar to the observation of all of the characteristics and qualities of a *drishti,* with the sense of insight we can examine all aspects of an idea to better understand it. For the Hershey's Kiss exercise, personal meaning might be be derived by using the sense of insight. Perhaps, the Kiss represents the sweetness of life, which is better savored by taking your time to cherish every moment.

If an idea is disturbing or unpleasant, perhaps being the objective observer will diffuse its power. On the other hand, one should not focus on a disturbing thought if it proves to be too uncomfortable. Learned relaxation through yoga can take many different paths. Always choose the path of self-kindness.

Learning to relax through yoga is a long and arduous journey that requires patience. Just like any long journey, it is important to take time to rest and reset, both physically and emotionally. The above discussion of the five senses and additional internal senses stresses the need to be mindful of the physical body, but taking time to digest the experience by using your sense of insight is critical. In that regard, it is best to find a position that allows you to forget about the physical body. The child's pose epitomizes such a position. It is a passive posture that diverts attention away from physical sensations to a heightened awareness of thoughts, emotions and feelings. Other passive positions of the body can be equally effective at promoting self-reflection, such as the supine spinal twist. It is during those times of physical release that the sense of insight is most keen. Periodic check-ins to emotions and feelings are important to evaluate what is working, which thoughts inspire, what speaks to you, and what honors the body. It is an unrealistic expectation to think that everything in yoga will feel good. Checking in is important to divert focus away from anything that causes physical or mental discomfort by modifying your practice. Similar to the intensification of the awareness of the other senses through a connection with the breath, the sense of insight is heightened by breathing into what is visible within. It is a way to dig down deep to appreciate the special person who is so very worthy of love, both by self and by others.

As an exercise to experience the sense of insight, close your eyes and bring your hands into *anjali mudra,* or prayer hands, and rest them on your forehead, the location of the third eye *chakra,* the energy center for insight. First, engage your sense of touch, noticing the feel of the hands resting on the forehead. Breathe deeply to heighten that sensation. Slowly push your palms apart while the fingetips remain in contact, thereby forming a ball-like shape. Imagine that you are holding a ball of energy in the form of light, in this case an indigo light, as the *ajna chakra* is assigned the color indigo, one of the seven colors of the rainbow. Experience the energy and warmth of your beautiful light. With each inhalation the sense of touch fades as the energy of the light intensifies. With each exhalation, the energy begins to be drawn inward into the third eye. Feel the beautiful indigo light of the third eye *chakra* progressively glowing brighter and brighter with each successive inhalation until the intensity of the light becomes so great that it begins to spread throughout the body. That wonderful indigo light represents your inner beauty. Feel its positive energy spread down the arms, the torso and legs and up to the crown of head *chakra,* the energy center for spirituality. Inhale deeply into your light, imagine now your whole body aglow with the wonderful indigo light of your inner beauty, and simply exhale into relaxation. Take a few moments to digest your experience.

Imagery is a wonderful way to engage your creativity to connect to your unique perceptions of the external world and the internal self. This exercise may have had a positive effect on your mood or allowed you to relax. At the very least, it brought your focus inward with a consideration of the human quality of inner beauty. It created an idea or a string of ideas on which to focus, ideas that existed in the moment.

The senses allow for the full experience of life, especially when focused upon individually. As you practice yoga, experiment with different points of focus, being deliberate with your choice. The possibilities are endless, such that your yoga practice need not ever be the same each time you arrive on your mat. The hope is that eventually you will no longer need to be deliberate in being mindful. You will become like a camera with autofocus that provides great clarity of all of the wonders of the marvelous world around you and the inner beauty within you.

8

THE LOVE OF WISDOM AND THE LOVE OF SELF

To be quite honest, if I am depressed or anxious, thinking about yogic philosophy is not high on my list. Further, one could argue that writings that are centuries old are no longer relevant to our modern day, high-tech, busy lifestyles and, even more so, to the main theme of this book, that is coping with mental illness. Of course, if that were the case, I could end this chapter right here. The beauty of philosophy, however, is that there are concepts that span the ages and, once embraced, provide for a broader understanding and a greater appreciation of our world and all it has to offer. Learned relaxation is an art and, as the artist, your palette can include beautiful words that come from a philosophy that defines life and the meaning of existence.

The word philosophy comes from the ancient Greek word *philosophia,* which translates to the "love of wisdom". My hope is that by embracing the philosophy of yoga, you can come to cherish its precepts to better understand yourself, affirm your worth and, ultimately, love yourself. A consideration of profound ideas that are advanced in the ancient Hindu scriptures and the teachings of the various yogic traditions to follow can lead to novel ways of thinking, with the power to alter pre-existing habitual thoughts and behaviors, broaden your perspectives of both yoga and life, and help overcome any challenges you face.

The following discussion is not meant to be an exhaustive, comprehensive exploration of all of yogic philosophy. I have attempted to dissect out the concepts that I feel are most applicable to an appreciation of yoga in the context of the themes of this book.

The oral traditions of yoga are felt to date back five millennia and were first written down in the Vedas and the Upanishads, the ancient, sacred Hindu religious texts, some three to four thousand years ago. But perhaps no one contributed more to the development of yoga as we know it today than Pantanjali, a sage believed to have lived circa 200 CE. *The Yoga Sutras,* his seminal treatise on the practice of yoga as a way of life, would serve as the foundation for all classical yoga to follow. His writings best embody and conceptualize the practice of yoga in the context of our modern day world. *Sutra* is the Sanskrit word for "string" or "thread". In *The Yoga Sutras,* these threads are short rules and aphorisms that are woven together into a system of ethics and philosophy.

Pantanjali described the ascent up Eight Limbs leading to a liberation from the material entanglement of this world and an internal purification for revealing the universal self. The Eight Limbs of Yoga are analogous to the rungs of a ladder that one climbs to reach the final limb of *samadhi,* the final step before enlightenment. It is the highest state of meditation in which one is fully absorbed without distraction in undisturbed contemplation and single-pointed concentration with the goal of attaining a full comprehension and understanding of every facet of the object of one's meditation. I certainly don't have an expectation to ascend to this highest limb, but I practice with the intent of clearing my mind to develop clarity as to how I wish to live my life and gaining insight into the qualities that constitute my true authentic self. I am positioned better to reduce distraction from thoughts that don't serve me, including regrets of the past, worries of the future, rumination on my suffering, and anxiety stemming from others' expectations that I feel I must live up to. The Eight Limbs of Yoga actually originally appeared in the *Upanishads,* however, it is through Pantajali's writings that this concept became more widely known. The Eight Limbs are a guide to living life to the fullest through a disciplined approach to yoga that can lead to states of inwardness and a connection to one's true passions and desires, while at the same time promoting deep states of relaxation and stress reduction.

The eight limbs are as follows:

Yamas ~ restraints

Niyamas ~ observances

Asanas ~ physical postures

Pranayama ~ breathing as a vehicle to balance *prana*, the life force

Pratyahara ~ the first state of introversion based on the flow of *prana*

Dharana ~ the initial stage of meditation arising from a single focus of concentration on a chosen object

Dhyana ~ the intermediate stage of meditation initiating the act of merging with the chosen object

Samadhi ~ the advanced and ultimate level of meditation devoid of distraction when the observer attains oneness with the object of observation and individual awareness dissolves

I like to think of the *yamas* and *niyamas* as analogous to the ten commandments. There are ten *yamas* and *niyamas,* five of each. Both the ten commandments and the *yamas* and *niyamas* represent tenets and principles that promote an ethical way of life, create moral standards in society and achieve long-lasting cultural strength and stability.

The *yamas* include:

- *ahimsa*, or non-harm
- *satya*, or truth
- *asteya*, or non-stealing
- *brahmacharya*, or restraint
- *aparigraha,* or non-possessiveness

The *niyamas* include:

- *saucha*, or purity and cleanliness
- *santosha*, or contentment

- *tapas*, or discipline
- *svadhyaya,* or the study of the self
- *Ishavara-Pranidhana,* or a devotion to what is greater than the self

Subjected to various interpretations throughout the ages, all of these concepts have numerous meanings and multiple layers of nuance. On a more global, cultural level, the *yamas* are restraints from what we should not do and the *niyamas* are observances that we should follow in order to lead an ethical life according to societal mores. On a more personal level, we can apply these principles to cope with the challenges that we face, including depression and anxiety.

An important proviso to keep in mind as you read on is that realistic expectations are necessary in order to gain the most benefit from an understanding of these philosophical principles. I am a practical person. I don't believe it would be useful for me to tell you that if you practice yoga and adhere to the *yamas* and *niyamas* life will improve and the challenges you face will disappear. From a practical perspective, however, a greater potential for self-realization might be possible through the practice of yoga in the context of the *yamas* and *niyamas.* Expectations are so important in attempting any endeavor. I might promote yoga as an avenue for self-discovery, but for many that may not occur. Non-attachment to outcomes is critical to enjoying the process. The best expectation is to expect nothing and just see how the process unfolds. For some, a dedication to a regular yoga practice may be spiritually life-changing. For others, it may just be a wonderful way to relax and rest from the stresses of life. My hope, of course, is that you will embrace yoga. Yoga is not just a series of movements and postures, but a philosophy by which to live. The principles of yogic philosophy have survived the ages. I believe that important words are long-lasting.

Ahimsa

As the first of the Pantanjali's Eight Limbs of Yoga, the *yamas* are the first step of the journey to a higher level of consciousness. The first of the five *yamas* is *ahimsa.* One meaning of *ahimsa* is nonviolence. Mahatma Gandhi was a strict adherent to this principle that became the core of his moral center. On a personal level, *ahimsa* also translates to non-harm. As we practice yoga with *ahimsa* we strive to neither harm body or mind. In ancient Hindu scriptures, when there is a list of terms, typically that which is mentioned first carries the greatest import. Such is true of *ahimsa,* the first of the *yamas. Ahimsa* represents the first and foremost principle of the first limb of yoga, and as such, becomes a prerequisite for achieving all that follows. The practice of *ahimsa* must be embraced before attempting to master the *asanas* or *pranayama* or having any hope of entering into the four meditative limbs. In other words, and to be blunt, if you don't approach yoga with self-kindness, don't bother to attempt to develop a meaningful, regular practice. You will set yourself up to fail. You must become a good friend to yourself if you want to have any expectation for success at yoga and, for that matter, any success in coping with depression and anxiety or anything else in life.

With regard to honoring the body, a dedication to the principle of *ahimsa* keeps us safe and prevents injury. Most of us have physical limitations and challenges. As we practice, we must listen to our bodies. If a movement causes pain or, quite simply, just doesn't feel good, modify your practice. Clouding the mind with thoughts of physical discomfort and any associated negative self-judgments arising from perceived limitations is antithetical to gaining mental clarity. One should never feel compelled to do everything the teacher or others might be doing. Our culture promotes a sense of competition with others and within ourselves. Yoga is not a grand competition, but rather your own personal experience with your own self-expression of movement. While comparing yourself to others, pushing yourself into sensations of discomfort or pain is reckless and leads to injury. Always practice yoga with an awareness of your edge. The edge is a point where discomfort arises. Once you determine your edge, ease off from it. Pain and the potential for injury arises from exceeding your edge. Over time with much patience, gradually your edge will shift as flexibility increases with consequent pride arising through acknowledgement of your progress.

In order to honor the mind with *ahimsa*, as it bears

repeating and I cannot stress enough, one must practice yoga with self-kindness. The hope is that self-compassion and an acceptance of limitations will generalize to all life experiences. The inner critic, the part of the psyche that constantly judges our actions, thoughts and emotions, wishes just the opposite. Negative self-judgments interfere with the positive outlook necessary to progress in your practice. Peace of mind is more attainable by making a choice to not engage with the inner critic. When the inner critic rears its ugly head, acknowledge its presence and substitute any negative thought with a positive one. It is always better to focus on what you can do, and not on what you can't. *Ahimsa* is all about practicing self-love and kindness. Once achieved, you might have greater empathy towards others and the battles they face against their inner critics. Yoga is a learning experience. Learn to recognize the unique person that you are and learn to love that person. Take advantage of all you can and cherish every moment. It all begins with love and kindness.

Satya

Satya is the Sanskrit word for truth. *Satya* is a restraint from lying and false representation. *Satya* is not just about lying to others, but also to oneself. Aspiring to become someone you think others want you to be, rather than living as your true authentic self can press down upon the spirit. Self-imposed constraints to conform to others' expectations can be a source of depression and anxiety. A yoga practice affords one the luxury of time for self-reflection in order to arrive at genuine choices for living life. And just as flexibility and balance develop over time, so does the ability to access feelings of inwardness and clarity in order to discover your own truth.

Asteya

Asteya is the Sanskrit word for non-stealing. As with many other yogic terms, *asteya* has many layers and meanings. In one sense, it refers to the restraint from stealing another's possessions or ideas or robbing precious resources from the Earth. *Asteya* can also refer to stealing time. We have only a limited time to be on this Earth. By becoming mired in regrets of the past and worries of the future, we are wasting precious time by letting all of the present moments pass by. Time can also be stolen away from the opportunity to practice self-care and build resiliency. The reality is that bouts of depression and anxiety can rob us of time spent in more productive pursuits. But quite simply, we can only do the best we can. Perhaps, a regular yoga practice might prevent mental illness from being that time thief.

Brachmacharya

In the ancient yogic tradition, *Brachmacharya* referred to the practice of celibacy and restraint from other worldly desires in order to redirect energy toward more enlightened, introverted states of being. More applicable to our modern times is a restraint from attaching to outcomes and, instead, staying in the moment to enjoy the process. Feelings of accomplishment from positive outcomes and successes in yoga are often fleeting. Attaching to the possibility of failure can reinforce pre-existing negative self-judgments and make self-fulfilling prophecies realities. A preoccupation with success comes with a fear of failure. The appreciation of the moment with disregard for outcomes leads to a greater chance of success without the pressure to perform, that is if we define success as becoming receptive to new possibilities that hold the potential for joy and contentment.

Aparigraha

Meaning non-possessiveness, *aparigraha* is the restraint from coveting and desiring material possessions, especially at the expense of others. It is a restraint from greed, pursuing only what is necessary for a modest life. In a sense, it is also being satisfied with what you have and, at the same time, not taking anything for granted. Similar to *brahmacharya*, embracing the principle of *aparigraha* promotes non-attachment to both material possessions and the potential outcomes of one's actions.

Non-attachment is one of the primary themes of the *Bhagavad Gita,* an ancient Hindu scripture written on the order of 2,200 to 2,500 years ago. The story centers on the great struggle between two branches of a single ruling family, the Kauravas and the Pandavas, and the personal struggles of the great warrior Arjuna, the leader of the Pandava army. Realizing that his enemies are his own relatives, cherished friends, and wise teachers, Arjuna is filled with doubt and sadness on the battlefield and refuses to fight. As the action of the battle freezes in time, Arjuna begins his analysis of what seemingly is a no-win situation. In hopes of solving his moral dilemma, he seeks out the advice of his charioteer, Lord Krishna, one of the principal Hindu deities and the god of love and compassion. Krishna urges Arjuna to practice non-attachment to the potential outcomes of the ensuing battle, even if they are tragic. Krishna explains to Arjuna that his path in life, or *dharma,* is as a warrior and prince. Despite his misgivings, he has a duty to be true to himself. His pre-destined role in this world necessitates that he enter into battle.

Non-attachment is a strategy of living without any expectations or self-imposed pressure to realize satisfaction from what we perceive lies only in our successes. Non-attachment is the acceptance of either possibility of success or failure and being content with either outcome. The mind becomes clouded by anxieties of the future, but clears with greater awareness of the present. Although final outcomes are secondary, arguably greater focus on the present moment may enhance performance and favor a successful outcome. In yoga, one should not attach oneself to goals of increased flexibility, introverted states or performing all of the postures perfectly. Rather, yoga should be a practice of enjoying the process. You can rest assure that with dedication, all of its benefits will follow.

The *Bhagavad Gita* also professes the value of connecting with one's true authentic self, as evinced by this quote, "Far better to live your own path imperfectly, than to live another's path perfectly." Internal conflict is inherent to the repression of our true desires and passions. Living a version of ourselves that we think others want us to be can result in emotional turmoil. And as Polonius so eloquently says to Laertes in *Hamlet,* "This above all – to thine own self be true". Whether consciously or subconsciously, denial of one's identity with regard to sexuality, gender, relationships and career, amongst many others, can generate mental friction. It is the concept of one's actual life purpose and path, or *dharma,* that lies at the heart of the *Bhagavad Gita.*

Dharma is a guiding principle in many Eastern religions. In Hinduism, *dharma* has multiple meanings, many without direct English translations. *Dharma* is considered the moral order of the universe. Another meaning pertains to living by a code of morality and adhering to principles advanced through law, religion and personal duty. It is behaving according to *Rta,* the order in the universe that gives rise to life. *Adharma,* the opposite of *dharma,* are behaviors and thoughts that are immoral and evil, resulting in discord and a disturbance in the universe. *Dharma* also refers to one's predestined true calling. In the *Bhagavad Gita,* Arjuna must live life as a warrior and adhere to those qualities that define a warrior. It is his identity and true purpose in life. Similar in thought is the expression, "Born to..." We often remark that someone was born to be a musician, an artist, a mathematician, etc. *Dharma also* applies to all beings on Earth; mammals, fish, insects, etc., which all possess predetermined life functions and behaviors. For many of us, finding one's *dharma* can be a lifelong pursuit.

The Sanskrit word *karma* translates to "action". Originally, *karma* in this life was thought to affect one's experience in the next. Today, the term is used more in terms of actions that affect future satisfaction and contentment in this life. Acting ethically, being morally principled and exhibiting behaviors that are rooted in altruism and kindness create so-called "good" *karma*. "Bad" *karma* results from malevolent behaviors, egocentrism, and evil intent, all potentially leading to pain and suffering for oneself and others.

As mentioned, part of living according to *aparigraha* is not taking anything or anyone for granted. It takes empathy and effort to assure others that you love and support them, and most importantly, are grateful for them. The hope of any meaningful relationship quickly fades when taking others for granted and behaving without respect or regard for their feelings; leading to estrangement at its worst.

Saucha

The first of the *niyamas, saucha* translates to purity and

cleanliness. It refers to the purity of body and mind that must be attained to develop a sense of well-being. In regard to the external purity of the body, *saucha* is achieved through daily washing, proper nutrition, restorative sleep and other forms of self-care.

Internal purity refers to a cleansing of the mind. An impure mind filled with anger, hate, greed, prejudice, and pride can be cleansed through yoga, meditation, and positive self-affirmations. Purity is realized by choosing to live with a positive perspective and kindness toward others. Purity of mind translates to self-love and compassion, which in turn gives one the capacity for love and compassion toward others. Just as we count negative numbers backwards, becoming mired in negativity draws us back from a calm and peaceful life. Instead, anger and hatred destroy the spirit and the life within us. Positivity allows us to progress toward a meaningful and profound life with satisfaction stemming from the wonderful effects you realize as you love and care for others, especially the gratitude you feel in return.

Santosha

Santosha is contentment, which can be realized through the practice of non-attachment. By not attaching ourselves to any desired goals, we can aspire to want what we have and not desire to have what we want. We try to practice yoga on and off the mat. Off the mat, acquiring material things may bring a sense of contentment, but that contentment may be fleeting. On the mat, attachment to the performance of an *asana* perfectly may set one up for failure and negative self-judgments. Even achieving that perfect posture ultimately may not give meaning to one's practice if not balanced with humility. It is interesting that contentment is one of the observances; what we should do. But, how do we "do" contentment? Perhaps, *santosha* can be realized through gratitude. In the Kripalu yogic tradition, we end our practice by saying, "Jai Bhagwan!", one definition of which is "a blessed victory." How one's practice is a victory is up to individual interpretation. For me, the contentment that comes from being grateful for all of the blessings of my life is a true victory!

Tapas

Tapas means "heat." It is also sometimes translated to "discipline." Like many yogic concepts, *tapas* can be interpreted many ways. One is the presence in the human spirit of a fiery passion, which through discipline can be harnessed to energize the spirit. Dedication and hard work are required to realize one's truth. When the practice of yoga is done with passion, its beneficial effects become more far-reaching. Desires for peace and contentment fuel a passion for yoga, the heat of *tapas*.

Svadhyaya

Svadhyaya is the fourth *niyama* that is the study or observation of self. Through yoga, we gain the capacity for introspection. Once again, we strive to create an authentic version of who we are. Conflict arises in the attempt to live up to someone else's expectation of whom we should be. Inner conflict is at the very least unsettling. In its extreme, it causes depression and anxiety, sometimes leading to desperate acts. The resolution of that inner conflict puts one on the path to peace and contentment. Practicing *svadhyaya* is easier said than done, but without attempting self-realization, the process of calming the mind can never begin. Inertia is only disturbed through the application of energy to change the course of a moving object; in this case the mind floating through a state of unhealthy inaction. Yoga can provide the spark for change and transformation.

Ishvara pranidhana

Ishvara pranidhana literally translates to, "devotion or surrender to the supreme being or God". A secular interpretation of *Ishvara pranidhana* is, "the humility that arises from the realization that one is only a minute part of an expansive universe." It is this larger perspective that diminishes the importance of self and individual inner conflicts stemming from issues of the ego. Egoism can be replaced by both an intellectual and emotional exploration of our miraculous world. We are only a small part of the wonders of nature and our planet. Moving away from anthropocentrism, *Ishvara pranidhana* becomes a devotion to the protection of all of the species on planet Earth. Whether one believes in a supreme being or not, our universe remains mysterious. What we experience and confront on a daily basis may represent fated events or random coincidences. Distinguishing between the two is arguably impossible. Practicing *Ishvara pranidhana* is gaining an acceptance that much exists that is beyond our ken, while at the same time not abandoning a pursuit of truth through inquiry. Nature in and of itself is awe-inspiring, full of miracles and beauty. The realization that we are a part of nature creates a oneness and connection between self and the world.

At the very least, a consideration of the *yamas* and the *niyamas* can be thought provoking. An active attempt to apply their principles requires work, but their implementation can change one's general outlook on life. They are a guide to self-realization that stresses honoring oneself with kindness, compassion and gratitude. They can serve as a wonderful framework on which to build a meaningful yoga practice. If one adheres to Pantanjali's model of the Eight Limbs of Yoga, embracing the *yamas* and *niyamas* will facilitate achieving states of inwardness with a purity of a mind free from toxic and disturbing thoughts.

From the principles of Classical Yoga put forth by Pantan-jali, other traditions arose, including Hatha yoga, which represents the main form of yoga that we practice today in the

Western world. The word *hatha* literally means "force". For the first time, Hatha yoga introduced the integration of the physical body, the breath and the mind. Much of the traditions of Hatha yoga come from the *Hatha Yoga Pradipika,* written in the 15th century by Svatmarama and based on the teachings of the 11th century, great sage Matsyendranath. As mentioned previously, according to Hindu mythology, Matysendranath, also known as the Lord of the Fishes, was given the secrets of Hatha yoga from the deity Shiva. Seeing an ominous star in the sky when Matysendranath was born, his parents threw him into the ocean where he was subsequently swallowed by a fish. At the bottom of the sea, Matsyendranath overheard god Shiva imparting the precepts of Hatha yoga to the goddess Parvati. For many years, Matsyendranath practiced his newfound knowledge of yoga inside the belly of the fish. He emerged twelve years later as an enlightened master of the practice of Hatha yoga. Gorakshanath, a later disciple of Matsyendranath, subsequently developed a new system of yogic rituals: *asanas, pranayama* and *dhyana,* or meditation.

The masters of Hatha yoga advanced the idea of a life force or *prana* that activates the subtle body. *Prana* is received into the body with the breath and then flows into the deeper self and spirit. Once *prana* is brought into the body from the external world, it then must be balanced. To that end, an anatomical system of energy centers and channels was proposed that facilitate the flow of *prana* throughout the body. The energy network not only establishes a healthy balance of *prana* throughout the body, but also rids the body of an undesirable form of energy called *apana*. Resiliency in the face of mental illness comes not only from accessing the life force through the control of the breath, but also from ridding the mind of unhealthy thoughts, thereby creating a balance that can smooth out variations in mood.

Some sources offer another definition of *hatha:* a compound word consisting of the word *"ha"* or sun and *"tha"* or moon. In a sense, the interplay of the physical and mental aspects of a Hatha practice energize the *pingala* and *ida nadis,* or the sun and moon energy channels, resulting in the complementary experiences of activity and heat and rest and cooling.

The main energy centers and channels in the body are known as *chakras* and *nadis,* respectively. Whether or not you believe in the actual existence of *chakras* and *nadis,* at the very least they can serve as useful metaphors, allowing one to imagine the flow of the energy of *prana* throughout the body. In addition, the ideas advanced by the ancient yogis are one of the earliest attempts to describe human anatomy and physiology. Many of their proposed ideas correspond to aspects of the nervous system as we know them today. One example is their knowledge that the left brain governs the right body and the right brain, the left, as evinced by their description of the decussation of the *ida* and *pingala nadis.* Another example is the sacral *chakra,* the energy center for sexuality and creativity, which is located in the region of our sacral plexus, which innervates our genitalia. Depending on the particular source cited, anywhere from 72,000 to 350,000 to millions of *nadis* in the body have been described. *Prana* also activates the seven main *chakras* and fuels *agni*, the fire burning in the belly. Again, considering this concept as a metaphor, *agni* might represent one's zeal and enthusiasm for life, both of which increase with the development of a more positive outlook.

The reported number of *chakras* also differs from text to text, but seven are the most commonly accepted number. The seven *chakras* are energy centers situated in the deep core of the body, the neck and head. The word *chakra* is Sanskrit for "wheel". Movements, directed thought and the breath can cause these wheels to spin. The *chakras* contain potential energy that becomes converted to the will, motivation and determination to better tackle life's challenges. From inferior to superior, they are the root, sacral, solar plexus, heart, throat, third eye and crown of head *chakras*. A regular yoga practice causes the "the wheels to spin" and creates the optimal balance between our body, mind and breath, thereby maximizing the influx of the lifeforce into the body.

Each of the *chakras* is assigned a particular color of the rainbow. Sir Isaac Newton observed that light passing through a prism is refracted or bent, emerging as the specific individual components of the spectrum of visible light. Although we now know that the visible spectrum of light is a continuous range of colors, he divided it into seven primary colors. ROYGBIV (red, orange, yellow, green, blue, indigo, and violet) is the traditional mnemonic that we were taught sometime in our schooling to aid in remembering those colors, which many of us still rely upon each time we marvel at the beauty of a rainbow. A rainbow is produced by a multitude of residual rain droplets suspended in the air that act as tiny prisms as the sun comes out after a storm, bending the sunlight into a beautiful arc of colors. The colors assigned to the seven *chakras* from inferior to superior range from red for the root chakra to violet for the crown chakra. Light is emitted in regular sine waves with peaks and troughs. The distance between two peaks of a wave is the wavelength. The shorter the wavelength, the more waves will occur in a given time and the higher the frequency of that light. Higher frequency light has greater energy. Therefore, violet light will have more energy than red light. Of course, ultraviolet light, which is just beyond the visible spectrum, has enough energy to be damaging to the skin with potential inducement of skin cancers. So keep in mind that as we proceed up through the seven *chakras*, the light energy associated with each one will possess incrementally greater energy than the preceding one as the frequency of light increases. This is fitting since the greatest energy lies in the high frequency violet light assigned to our crown *chakra*, the center of our spirituality. What a beautiful image of the energies of the soul that make up our unique personalities, all aglow with the colors of the rainbow. Your own glowing light illuminates the path to self-realization. Others will see that light in your expressions of love and compassion.

Returning back to the theme of this book, mindfulness of

the moment to elicit feelings of relaxation, existing in that moment are thoughts that arise from directed focus on physical sensations, as well as any idea, whether concrete or abstract. Whether you believe in the existence of the *chakras* or they are just useful metaphors, deliberate thought directed at their activation, causing the wheels to spin, and their associated deep, profound meanings exist in the moment. Each *chakra* is assigned different attributes, energies and power. Some of their meanings may resonate more with you than others. Personalizing their meanings elicits emotions that are heightened by breathing deeply into the location of each *chakra*. Ideas represented by the *chakras* include safety, creativity, wisdom, love and compassion, expression, insight and spirituality, among others.

The seven *chakras* from inferior to superior in location:

Muladhara or Root Chakra

Assigned the color red, it is located between the sitz bones and the perineum, the inferior most border of the pelvis and the site of our genitals and anus, possessing the energy that grounds us to the earth. It is a reminder that we are part of this planet and have a deep responsibility to treat the environment and nature with compassion and respect. Its energy also creates a sense of safety, diminishing, anxiety, fear and anger, which are felt to be part of *apana* centered in the pelvis. In addition, the energy of the *muladhara chakra* fuels our passion for living.

Swadhisthana or Sacral Chakra

Assigned the color orange, it fuels our sexuality and creativity and lets us experience the joy from both. Our sexuality stems from our primitive urges that promote survival. Similarly, our creativity also developed to allow our species to flourish. Humans' creativity led to inventions such as tools and the wheel that significantly improved the abilities to hunt and farm.

Manipura or Solar Plexus Chakra

Above the root and sacral *chakras* lies the solar plexus or *manipura chakra*, assigned the color yellow. The solar plexus is located just above the navel and below the sternum and is called such because it represents a complex network of nerves in the abdomen that radiate out from a central point. Within that center is the energy that fuels our inner strength and wisdom. Inner strength is needed to face personal challenges. Wisdom leads to clarity, awareness and strategies for coping.

Anahata or Heart *Chakra*

We wish to balance the energies of all of our *chakras,* but arguably the most important *chakra* for contentment and peace is the *anahata* or heart *chakra.* It is the energy of our love, compassion and gratitude. Love and compassion for one's fellow beings, both human and otherwise, is a source of positive energy. Negative energy arises from conflict, grudges, judgments and criticisms. The close companion of love and compassion is gratitude. We can experience gratitude to the greatest degree at our heart center. Gratitude is one of the most powerful emotions that we can express as it is a prerequisite for all other positive emotions that we feel. Right now, connect to your *anahata chakra* by resting prayer hands in *anjali mudra* on the heart. Heartbeats that represent life are transmitted through the chest wall to pulsate the hands. It is felt that the energy of the heart center exits the body through the palms. In a sense, with the palms together, you might imagine creating an ever-growing revolving positive energy loop of love, compassion and gratitude.

Vishuddha or Throat *Chakra*

Assigned the color blue, it is this energy center that governs our ability to communicate. Therein lies our expression of our thoughts and feelings. Outward expressions of love, compassion and gratitude help others in need. Conversely, expressing one's feelings in an understandable way is necessary for an empathetic friend to know how to best support you in your time of crisis or need.

Ajna or Third Eye Chakra

We will never fully comprehend the miracles of life, however, it is our third eye or *ajna chakra,* assigned the color indigo, that allows us to have a keen awareness of the world. The third eye, located just above the bridge of the nose, is the portal to our higher consciousness and, through insight, can help us along our path to enlightenment. Our two eyes allow us to see the external world. The third eye sees beyond the physical. It perceives the energies of all that surrounds us, especially those of other living beings. Perhaps more importantly, the third eye can see inward, allowing for self-reflection and a connection to one's passions.

Sahasrara or Crown of Head Chakra

Finally, located above all other *chakras* in the body is the crown of head *chakra* or *sahasrara chakra,* assigned the color violet. This *chakra* contains the energy for our spirituality. We use that term often, but what exactly is meant by spirituality? One definition is, "the connection of the mind and soul to the external universe that transcends the physical world." An alternative definition is, "the driving force of life fueled by the incorporation of ideas and emotions into our experiential thinking."

The site of this *chakra* at the top of our head is fitting, since by climbing up the ladder of the *chakras* we have gone from the earth at our root to the universe above our crown of head. This direction of flow is known as the energy of liberation. The reverse flow toward the earth is known as the energy of manifestation. One flow of energy frees us from earthly stresses in order to find spiritually. The other energy flow determines how we manifest as unique people on earth. We can experience the energy flow of liberation in our yoga practice by creating lines of energy extending from the earth, through the legs, up the spine and out the crown of the head into the heavens. The universe is vast, but we are all a vital part of it.

As we develop a meaningful practice, accessing and balancing the energy of the *chakras* will allow us to feel grounded and safe, in touch with our sexuality and creativity, wise and strong, loving and compassionate, powerful through self-expression, in awe of the miracles and blessings of the world around us and within us, and spiritually connected to the universe. The rainbow of the colors of the *chakras* emerges as the storm of inner conflict is calmed and the sunlight of clarity emerges. Through the practice of yoga, we receive *prana,* the life force. Metaphorically speaking, *prana* might be considered the meaning derived from the often hidden blessings that surround us all.

The practice of yoga can be a vehicle for personal growth

through an analysis and exploration of one's personal belief system coupled with a willingness to change. It is important to understand that yoga is so much more than the physical postures. Connecting the postures to their meanings and symbolisms elevates one's experience.

To derive the most benefit from the study of the philosophy of yoga, it is necessary to find practical applications in abstract ideas. As a yoga instructor, I embraced the traditions of Kripalu yoga, a practical philosophy that makes many of the ancient tenets of yoga relevant to our modern day. I was drawn to its philosophy, which promotes the idea of inclusiveness regardless of physical limitations or mental challenges. I learned that yoga isn't about being good or bad, it is just about being. Connecting with the true self that lies deep in the soul is the heart of Kripalu Yoga. One definition of the Sanskrit word *kripalu* is "compassion". Quite simply, Kripalu yoga is the practice of self-kindness and compassion. It is letting go of preconceived ideas, expectations and attachments to allow for the natural unfolding of one's experience. It is freedom from negative self-judgments and inner criticisms in the pursuit of clarity of mind. Kripalu yoga is a type of Hatha yoga that integrates the principles of classical yoga, including Pantanjali's Eight Limbs of Yoga, and blends ideas and concepts dating back to the ancient Vedic scriptures with modern day attitudes and practices. It professes an integration of movement, breathing and meditation to achieve self-actualization.

Arguably, the most important principle of the Kripalu

philosophy is "self-observation without judgment." I can choose to simply observe my physical abilities and limitations in assuming an *asana* without qualifying them. It is being fine with who you are without desiring to be someone you're not. If I an unable to be steady in a balance posture, two thoughts may arise. One is, "I am wobbling or falling out of the pose." The second is, "I will never be able to balance." The first statement is an observation. The second is a judgment. The second statement serves no purpose other than feeding the inner critic. As you practice yoga, take time to reflect on your thoughts. Notice what are observations and what are judgments. Negative judgments are more often cognitive distortions. Once you notice that you are judging yourself, dispel the myth of your distortion of reality and give yourself a break to just be satisfied with who you are. In order to dispel the myth of the above example, rather than telling yourself that you won't ever be able to balance, tell yourself that the potential exists that with practice I might be able to better achieve physical balance or it is alright and rather inconsequential if I have trouble assuming a balance posture. Better than jumping to the false, negative conclusion of failure is practicing non-attachment to final outcomes and being aware of the process. In fact, you might even enjoy your wobbling. As a teacher, I often wonder if students in my class would find more difficulty in being told to wobble than to sustain a balance posture in stillness, and at the same time having fun doing it.

In essence, "self-observation without judgment" is synonymous with the practice of self-kindness. There is always the potential for two people to show up on your mat. One is self-critical, beating you up with negativity and leaving you in a mental and emotional state of exhaustion. The other is kind, proud of your accomplishments, and respectful of your limitations. Think about how you would treat someone on the adjacent mat. Would you criticize them or, with kindness, be a supportive friend. Be that good friend to yourself. The choice of who shows up on your mat is yours and, as such, in your full control.

Although I have tried to embrace the many principles of yogic philosophy, it is gratitude that guides me most. For those with mental disease, positive emotions can be elusive. A useful exercise to connect with feelings of gratitude is done by pausing, closing the eyes, creating an image in your mind of someone or something you are grateful for, and then taking a deep breath into that image. I often breathe into the gratitude I have for the support of the loved ones in my life and the realization that they are equally grateful for me.

A philosophy is most impactful if its principles have practical applications to daily life. The teachings of yogic philosophy exist on many different levels. More globally, they are a set of rules to bind a society with ethical and moral expectations. More personally, they provide the path to authenticity; living according to your *dharma,* your true purpose. Most importantly, they possess valuable knowledge for living in contentment and peace that begins with self-kindness and gratitude. This wisdom is a treasure that, when embraced, possesses the power to better understand your essence. The wisdom of philosophy becomes wisdom of the self. The hope is that from the latter, you will recognize the unique individual you are; worthy of love from others and, most importantly, from yourself.

It is now time to move on from the theoretical to the practical. The exploration of the breathing and postural techniques of yoga to follow will serve as the foundation for your practice of relaxation, providing you with practical tools to assuage the deleterious effects of depression and anxiety. Up until this point, I have presented the many sides of yoga in the context of coping with depression and anxiety. An awareness of the scope of your mental challenges, your physiological responses to stress, the benefits of yoga to your body and mind, your experience of being mindful of sensations, and your newfound wisdom of self all possess the power to generate ideas that pertain to what you are doing in the present moment. Being in the moment is at the heart of learned relaxation. My hope is that you will embrace all that yoga has to offer to not just live in the moment, but to cherish every moment.

PART II

THE PRACTICE OF LEARNED RELAXATION

9

STRETCHING INTO RELAXATION

The following chapters are meant to present you with the tools to achieve learned relaxation that I believe are more effective in the context of newfound knowledge that I hope you accrued in the first part of this book. The practice of yoga opens us up to new perspectives and possibilities by offering us a whole array of sensations, ideas, thoughts and emotions on which to focus. Individualizing your practice is a process of so-called "picking and choosing" that which has the greatest impact on your ability to relax and, most importantly, to cope with whatever challenges you face. You might think of the second part of this book as an extensive menu of different ways to approach your yoga, some which may speak to you more than others. Ultimately, my hope is that you can create your own palette of profound ideas in order to fully embrace the art of learned relaxation.

Unlike other forms of meditation, yoga possesses a physicality that can become the object of single-pointed concentration. As mentioned previously, as we transition from pose to counterpose, antagonistic muscles alternately stretch and contract. As contraction abates, muscular tension is released, which through deliberate, directed awareness can translate into a release of mental stress. Release can then turn into pleasure by actively stretching a muscle. Quite simply, stretching muscles feels good. On a more complex, physiological basis, feelings of release and pleasure can stimulate the parasympathetic nervous system and perhaps initiate the release of "happy hormones." In essence, we are stretching into relaxation.

Yoga affords a unique opportunity to enjoy a physical experience that is formally organized into a system of poses, or *asanas*, that can be used to quiet an active mind. The traditionally performed *asanas* that comprise that system serve as a common ground on which practitioners can learn and instructors of yoga can teach. *Asana* is a Sanskrit word that translates to "position" or "posture". In reality, any position of the body could be considered an *asana*. And of course, any series of movements connected to the breath on which to meditate constitutes yoga; the integration of body, breath and mind.

The *asanas* are an important component of learned relaxation. Self-reflection and the experience of physical sensations are done in the present moment. Being in the present clears the mind of rumination on the past and future that can cloud the mind with stress and negativity.

As you practice yoga on a regular basis, there is potential for the *asanas* to become too familiar and habitual. Muscle memory obviates the need for deliberate thought to enter into a particular posture. Familiarity can allow the mind to wander. Mind chatter increases and stress levels can rise. Small changes in the positioning of body parts or small movements to convert static postures into more dynamic fluid ones introduce novelty into your practice. Novelty engages the mind. A small bend in one finger while in warrior pose or a slight swaying of the hips in mountain directs all focus to these small variations that are occurring in the present moment. By becoming mindful of these minor changes in the body, the mind no longer has an opportunity to wander.

The *asanas* are more than just specific ways to position the body in space. Each one is an opportunity for self-expression. Each one can elicit novel thoughts through symbolism and historical references, especially when experienced in the context of personal meaning. Through focused, deliberate thought, you possess the power to transform any *asana* into a profound experience, imbued with the energy needed to change your perspectives and outlook for the better.

The following discussion illustrates how an *asana* can take on a life of its own through personal reflection and an appreciation of the experience of the physical body. For this exercise, find a peaceful and quiet place where you can minimize any distractions. I recommend being barefoot on either a yoga mat or a hard, firm floor. Yoga is best done barefoot both to prevent slippage and to better and directly feel the bottoms of the feet grounding into the mat. Your feet are just like your hands. They are meant for gripping and exploring the world through the sensation of touch. Just as you wouldn't do yoga with gloves on, take your socks off.

For this exercise, we will explore *tadasana,* or the mountain pose. The mountain pose is the foundation for all of the standing postures. It promotes good posture through the elongation of the spine and engagement of the muscles of the core. At the same time, we experience a strong sense of the ground, connecting us with the supportive, firm earth below. It is a posture full of positive energy that boosts self-esteem as we stand strong and tall. *Tadasana* is a posture to honor the spine. As the main energy centers and pathways are thought to be intimately associated with the spine, it is also an important spiritual symbol of yoga.

Before assuming *tadasana,* let's consider what a mountain might represent. It certainly is a symbol of strength. It has a large base that grounds it to the earth, and its peak majestically reaches toward the heavens. It might also represent a daunting challenge for those who wish to scale it. To face that challenge we must be deliberate and disciplined as we climb. As we start our journey, the sheer height prevents us from seeing the summit. We must have faith that our goal is attainable even though it is not visible or fully known to us. Along our climb we will tire and may not want to continue, but as we rest we remind ourselves of our goal of reaching that summit, and then resume our quest. What new knowledge will we acquire and what emotions will we feel when we attain our goal? As we get closer to the very top of the mountain, our climb becomes more arduous. It is at this point that we must dig deep within to access more energy. The energy we need is what in yogic philosophy is known as *prana*. *Prana* is the life force. We must bring *prana* into our bodies and minds. *Prana* is all around us, but we must internalize it to come to know contentment and peace. Our source of *prana* is the breath. With each step up the slope, we concentrate more and more on the breath. We listen to its sound and feel the sensation of the breath entering and exiting the nose. We become aware of the rhythmic expansion of the chest, as the intercostal muscles between our ribs stretch and relax. Life-giving oxygen fuels our muscles. Heightening our focus on what is happening in the body helps us to enjoy the moment while not regretting any previous missteps along our journey or worrying about what lies ahead.

When we finally accomplish our goal, we can thoroughly enjoy our experience at the top of that strong, towering mountain. From the summit, we obtain a different perspective of the world around us. We can gain clarity of our true selves, our vision no longer blocked by the trees or rocks that once lined our path. We are closer to the stars scattered across the infinite universe. We realize that we are part of something more expansive and larger than ourselves. Problems that seemed so monumental now look so very small from up high. We salute both the light of the nurturing sun and our own light that has been ignited by our profound intention.

After consideration of the personal meanings and symbolism of *tadasana,* we can now layer on the physical aspects of the posture. From a health and wellness perspective, strengthening the spine is paramount as we age. There are deep paraspinous muscles that run the length of the spine. Picture those muscles as silly putty stuck to the posterior or back of the vertebrae. As those muscles contract, they pull the vertebrae back, bringing us upright. As we age, those muscles lose tone and muscle mass and we lose that posterior pull. Consequently, the spinal column begins to round forward. Unfortunately, in extreme cases, many people are left kyphotic or chronically bent over.

All *asanas* are built from the ground up, so for *tadasana* we must first root ourselves into the earth. Having a stable base leads to better balance and more effective engagement of the muscles of the body. Of course, for a standing posture, our base is our feet. So begin by placing the feet parallel and hip distance, or approximately six to eight inches, apart. As you stand, feel your weight evenly distributed on all parts of the feet, from the toes to the balls to the heels. Your feet, the mat and the earth are now all in continuity, becoming one.

Next, engage the muscles of your legs. Imagine that you are pushing your feet into the earth. Contract your leg muscles as if you are holding a block between your thighs. Engaging your thigh muscles, specifically your quadriceps muscles, will cause your kneecaps to rise up. The quadriceps muscles might feel as if they are wrapping around your femurs, the long thighbones. The legs are now both like strong tree trunks with the feet becoming like roots extending into the earth.

The pelvis is next on the ascent up our mountain. Consider the pelvis as a large bowl that anatomically angles downward from the sacroiliac joints in the back to the pubis in the front. Imagine that there is water filling the bowl of the pelvis. In order to prevent the water from spilling out over the front edge, it is necessary to drop the tailbone and raise the pubic bone; the bone is located about six inches below the navel. We don't want any waterfalls on our mountain. By dropping the tailbone, the normal curve or lordosis of the lumbosacral spine lessens, resulting in a more straight and longer lower spine.

With regard to the spine, there are seven cervical, twelve thoracic, five lumbar, five sacral vertebrae and the coccyx. The coccyx, usually composed of four segments at the very bottom of the spine, is the vestige of a tail that disappeared some time in evolution. The vertebrae of the sacrum are fused to add stability to the pelvis, but the other vertebrae more superiorly are capable of independent, although somewhat limited movements. Each vertebra articulates with other vertebrae, one below and one above, through the facet joints. The facet joints are located behind the spinal canal, the space in which lies the spinal cord. They are synovial joints that allow for movement of the spine in six directions that are incorporated into all yoga poses: forward, back, laterally to the right and left and twisting to the right and left. In front of the spinal canal, the round bony bodies of the vertebrae are separated from their neighbors by the intervertebral discs. The disc functions as a cushion to axial compressive forces on the spine. The intervertebral disc has a pliable, gelatinous substance centrally, the nucleus pulposis, surrounded by supportive, stronger and more firm tissue, the annulus fibrosus. Think of the intervertebral discs as shock absorbers between the vertebral bodies.

Our spines are also not straight vertical structures. They have curves or lordoses. In the laws of physics, a curved or arched structure can offer more resistance to axial loading forces relative to a straight one. The cervical lordosis is convex anteriorly or toward the front of our bodies, the thoracic lordosis convex posteriorly or toward the back, and the lumbar and sacral lordosis convex anteriorly. Since the sacral vertebrae are fused, we cannot alter the sacral lordosis. We can only vary the angulation of it in relation to the lumbar spine above. The goal in maximizing length in the spine is the decompression or stretching of the intervertebral discs and the distraction or opening up of the facet joints, both of which result in the elongation of the spine. The elongation then partially straightens the different segmental lordoses. The end result is a person standing straight and tall.

Let the arms be at your sides for now. In *tadasana,* although we try to emulate that strong mountain, the shoulders remain soft. If the shoulders move up towards the ears, the neck muscles contract and shorten the cervical spine. First, try scrunching your shoulders up to your ears. Notice your neck muscles engaging. Now release the shoulders and let the shoulder blades melt down your back. As they do, notice how much more the neck and cervical spine can lengthen in the opposite direction. The other secondary effect of letting the shoulders drop down the back is a movement of the sternum or breastbone up and forward, as if you are about to salute the general. With dropped shoulders, fingertips can be pulled away from the body in order to engage the arm muscles, further adding to the strength of your mountain. The final step is to subtly drop the chin towards the chest.

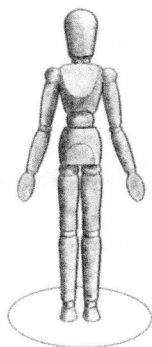

Tadasana ~ The Mountain

Congratulations! You are now standing strong and tall like a mighty mountain!

The arms can now be positioned anyway that is meaningful to you or just feels good. Wherever they might be positioned, the shoulders remain soft. By simultaneously engaging the muscles of the arms and legs, the muscles of the core are secondarily activated. Except for the relaxation of the shoulders and the facial muscles, the entire body is active and working. The arms can be angled down at the sides, palms facing forward, and fingers spread wide, as if one is receiving the life force of *prana* from the universe of which we are all a part. Spreading the fingers wide engages the forearm muscles. Alternatively, the hands might come together at heart center in *anjali mudra* as you take a moment to create an image in the mind of someone for whom you are grateful.

All that remains for the full expression of the *asana* is to breathe deeply into the stretch of the body. One might imagine a long line of positive energy has formed, coursing from the earth, up both legs and spine and shooting out through the crown of the head into the heavens above.

As you can see from the aforementioned exploration of *tadasana*, there is much to be discovered in the exploration of an *asana*, especially any personal meaning that lies at the heart of the pose, manifest as emotions and novel thoughts. Yoga that makes each *asana* one's own expression of self is a component of a type of yoga known as *viniyoga*, a practice performed to honor the needs of the individual; allowing for introspection and the uncovering of profound meaning in each *asana*.

Common to all of the *asanas* is that they all rise from the ground up, involve engagement and release of muscle groups particular to that posture, and result in balance; the balance of the body relative to the force of gravity and the balance of the body relative to the forces of the mind. It is in the latter that lies the power of yoga.

The remainder of this chapter is not meant to be a complete list and description of all of the *asanas*, or necessarily how to do them all. I do touch on thirty-one of the more common poses, some that can be referenced to Hindu scriptures or mythology, those that have personal meaning for myself and most that are used in the posture sequences in the next chapter. My discussion highlights a few of the choices on an extensive menu of profound ideas that can each serve as the object of your focus as you relax into each moment. My hope is that this discussion might provide you with some new perspectives that might promote self-inquiry into your yoga practice.

In addition, the choice of charcoal art figurines to illustrate the *asanas* was intentional. As alluded to previously, what attracted me to Kripalu yoga was the guiding principle of self-observation without judgment. I believe there is a tendency to compare oneself to the models in photographs doing each yoga pose. I will admit that when I see an extremely fit and flexible young person in a photograph seemingly fully comfortable in an *asana*, I am often guilty of envy. Potential also can exist for comparisons and negative self-judgments arising from one's poor body image. Even if I used so-called "average-appearing people" of varying body types and flexibility, I believe comparison is inevitable. So I choose to use illustrations that do not possess any emotional power or potential for self-judgments so that you can devote more of your attention to my words and less to thoughts that don't serve in the moment.

Utkatasana

The Chair Pose

The Sanskrit word *utkata* has many meanings including "powerful", "proud" and "fierce". The English name of this posture simply reflects the appearance of sitting in a chair, an imaginary one in this instance.

The name of this *asana* has its origin in Hindu mythology from the *Ramayana,* an epic poem written several thousands of years ago.

It follows the struggles of Rama, a divine prince from the Kosala Kingdom, following his exile from the kingdom by his father, King Dasharatha. With courage and strength, he overcomes many struggles and challenges as he travels across the Indian subcontinent with his wife, Sita, and brother, Laksh-

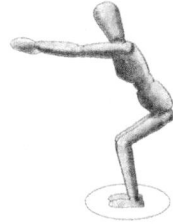

Utkatasana ~ The Chair Pose

mana. After fourteen years in exile, Rama returns to his birthplace, Ayodhya, to be crowned king and assume his rightful place on the throne.

The main theme of the myth is *utkata;* the power, courage, and ferocity embodied by Rama. As you assume *utkatasana,* you might consider a throne as a type of chair reserved for the powerful. As such, as you create your throne you might experience the power of positive affirmations and gratitude. Yoga provides an opportunity to connect with our true selves and passions, allowing us to embrace life. Tapping into that power can be quite liberating. Allow *utkatasana* to be more than just an imaginary chair, but rather a symbol of your pride that is realized through your yoga practice. Be proud of your courage in the battle to overcome whatever challenges you face.

Virabhadrasana
The Warrior

There are three distinct warrior poses in a typical Hatha yoga practice: warriors I, II and III. Warrior III is an advanced balance posture, but I will touch on it nonetheless so you can have a full appreciation of all three.

It always seemed odd to me that a peaceful practice like yoga that stresses *ahimsa,* or nonviolence, should incorporate a pose called the warrior. The origins of all three warrior poses, however, come from ancient Hindu mythology through a story of violence, revenge, remorse, sorrow, compassion and love. The symbolism of that myth embodies the *asanas* we do today.

The powerful King Daksha, father of Sati, disapproves of his daughter's marriage to Shiva, one of the principal deities of the Hindu religion and known as the Destroyer and Transformer. The King does not care for the reclusive god Shiva who meditates on mountain tops rather than being an active part of society. He also knows of Shiva's history of questionable behaviors, such as the decapitation of one of the five heads of Brahma, another one of the three principal Hindu deities.

King Daksha hosts a *yagna*, a religious sacrifice and celebration to which he invites all beings of heaven, except Shiva and his daughter, Sati. An enraged and slighted Sati goes to the *yagna* anyway. There, through her yoga, she enters into a deep state of meditation and rage, which fuels her inner fire to such a degree that it totally consumes her physical body. Hearing of his wife's tragic demise, Shiva rips off his clothes and tears out his hair. One of his torn locks is transformed into the malevolent warrior Virabhadra. Shiva instructs Virabhadra to go to the *yagna*, kill everyone there, behead the king and then drink his blood.

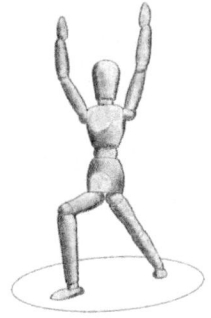

Virabhadrasana I ~ Warrior I

Virabhadra enters the *yagna* chest forward with two swords, one in each hand, raised above his head. Virabhadra's initial posture becomes *virabhadrasana* I, in which the hips and chest are squared forward with arms raised above the head and the front knee bent forward, poised to attack.

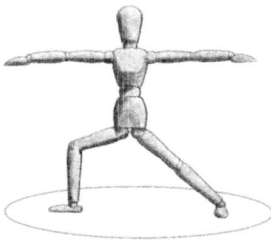

In *virabhadrasana* II, with an unwavering gaze directed over an extended sword in his front hand and his front knee bent forward into a lunge, he is ready to thrust the sword into the king.

Virabhadrasana II ~ Warrior II

Finally, in *virabhadrasana* III, the body becomes extended parallel to the ground with both arms extended forward next to the ears while balancing on one leg. It is as if Virabhadra is holding two swords directed downward, ready to kill the king lying beneath him. Balancing on one leg symbolizes his final commitment to drive the swords through the neck of the king.

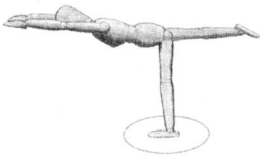

Virabhadrasana III ~ Warrior III

After Virabhadra kills the king and everyone else at the celebration, Shiva arrives and witnesses all of the death and destruction for which he was responsible. With great remorse and compassion he absorbs Virabhadra back into his body and restores life back to everyone, including King Daksha. Sati, his wife, is reincarnated as Parvarti, the goddess of fertility, marriage, strength, devotion and power.

The meanings and messages of this myth are up to individual interpretation. One might reflect on the importance of restraint in order to avoid the remorse and sorrow that may result from rash and reflexive actions in emotionally charged situations. More importantly, all of the warrior poses afford an opportunity to consider how each of us is a proud warrior in life, having overcome

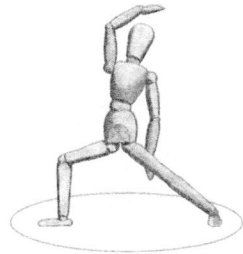

Viparita Virabhadrasana ~ Reverse Warrior

or presently facing life's challenges with determination and courage.

From warrior II, the front arm can be swept up and overhead into *Viparita virabhadrasana,* the Reverse Warrior, with the spine twisted to open up the chest to the sky, as if you are receptive to the vast power of the universe that can then empower you to face your own challenges.

Baddha Virabhadrasana
The Humble Warrior

One enters into this *asana* from warrior I. Hands can be brought into *anjali mudra* at heart center as one bows forward from the hip creases.

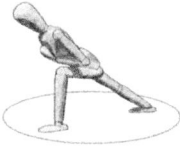

The Humble Warrior

In response to upper body weight shifting forward as you bend, deliberate grounding into both feet equally is necessary to maintain balance and lower body strength. A humble warrior needs to be well grounded.

A meaningful yoga practice is approached with humility and modesty with a de-emphasis on the importance of personal success. Being humble is not attaching to either success or failure, but being satisfied with either outcome. Gaining control over feelings of depression and anxiety through one's yoga practice is a true personal victory. Success, however, is not a prerequisite to experience pride. Rather, pride can be felt in recognizing all of the work done in any attempt to achieve your goal, regardless of the outcome.

Trikonasana

The Triangle Pose

The sides of a triangle connect to each other. There are many different classifications of triangles based on the lengths and relationship of the three sides and the value of each of the three angles formed.

An equilateral triangle has three congruent sides and angles. It is balanced in its symmetry. An isosceles

Trikonasana ~ The Triangle Pose

triangle has two congruent sides and two congruent angles. A right triangle possesses one right or ninety degree angle. The relationship of its three sides is described by the Pythagorean theorem. Pythagoras was an ancient Greek philosopher who was the first to articulate this relationship centuries ago. As we assume *trikonasana,* we create two adjacent triangles. One triangle formed by our two legs and the mat connects us to the earth, instilling in us a sense of safety. The other triangle formed with our front leg, arm and torso connects us to ourselves. Therein lies the power of yoga.

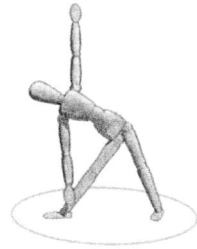

Utkata Konasana

The Goddess Pose

This *asana* is about harnessing the power, pride and ferocity of a goddess. The goddess embodies the femininity of *ida,* the moon energy channel, coupled with the active masculine characteristics of *pingala,* the sun energy channel.

While in the goddess pose, one might consider *Tridevi,* the three principal goddesses of Hinduism:

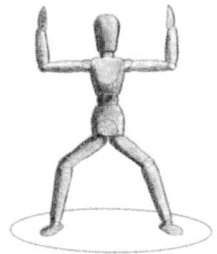

Utkata Konasana ~ The Goddess Pose

1. Saraswati, the wife of Brahma and the goddess of learning, arts and music.
2. Lakshmi, the wife of Vishnu and the goddess of fortune and wealth.
3. Parvati, the wife of Shiva and the goddess of fertility, marriage, strength, devotion and power.

With regard to Parvati, she embodies *shakti,* or the primordial energy of the universe. Parvati created Ganesha, the ruler over all beings, both earthly and celestial, and the remover of all obstacles. One story recounts that Ganesha was created by his mother, Parvati, using earth that she molded into a boy. While Parvati's husband, Shiva, was away, Parvati charged her new son with guarding the cave while she bathed. Upon his return home, Shiva is met by Ganesha who bars his entry into the cave. Upon hearing Ganesha's claim as the son of Parvati, Shiva is outraged and cuts off his head. Parvati is devastated by the death of her son. Feeling remorse, Shiva searches for a new head for the boy. As the first animal he saw was an elephant, Ganesha is depicted as a human form with an elephant's head.

As we practice the goddess pose, perhaps we can tap into the strength of Ganesha, in the hopes of removing any obstacles to peace and contentment. And with regard to mental challenges, our hope is to become the goddess of harmony and happiness.

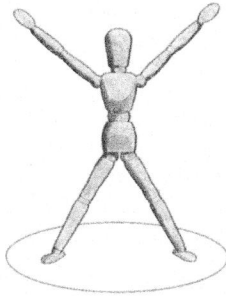

Utthita Tadasana
The Star Pose

Utthita Tadasana ~ The Star Pose

A star is the creator of life. Without its warmth and light, all life would not be able to thrive. Depression and anxiety often prevent us from thriving. The intention of the star pose is to generate your own warmth and light to provide the energy to take action, even if it is taking on the simplest of tasks.

By energizing the heart center with thoughts of love, compassion and gratitude, like the energy that emanates from the center of a star, heat and warmth will spread out throughout your body and beyond. The stretching of the arms and grounding of the feet serve as four lines of energy that ignite the inner light of your star for everyone to see.

Garudasana

The Eagle Pose

Garuda is the king of the birds in Hindu mythology, as well as in Buddhism and Jainist lore. He is the avian protector of the Hindu god Vishnu, able to transport him anywhere he wishes to go.

As one enters *garudasana,* an intimacy develops with one's body that is experienced as the arms and legs become intertwined. Right and left become one as one focuses on and observes a single *drishti* in order to achieve physical balance. The *ida nadi* that channels the energy of the right brain and left nostril and body and the *pingala nadi* that channels the opposite sided energy come into balance. Heat balances cooling, impulsiveness balances rational thought, and the feminine and masculine energies become one. One might imagine vertical lines of energy that extend through all four limbs that are bent and crisscross in front of the body.

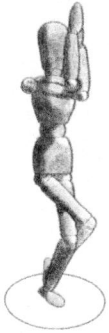

Garudasana ~ The Eagle Pose

All of the *asanas* are open to individual interpretation. Yoga provides us with this wonderful opportunity for innovative thought and self-exploration. The art of learned relaxation requires a connection with one's individuality, expression and imagination, with the potential for personal growth. Tapping into one's creativity lets the spirit soar like an eagle!

Vrikshasana

The Tree Pose

One might imagine themselves a tree. Many species of trees exist, like the strong oak, the graceful weeping willow and the energetic aspens with their quivering leaves, to just name a few.

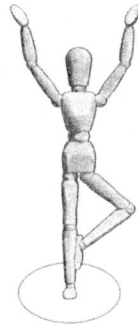

Vrikshasana ~ The Tree Pose

As yoga is a personal experience and you are a unique thinker, the image in the mind of the type of tree that suits you best can serve as another point of focus, which along with your *drishti*, can facilitate physical balance.

You might build upon your mind's image by considering

the standing leg as the strong trunk of your tree and the outstretched arms as the branches that represent the myriad facets of your personality molded by life experiences and the inherent qualities that make you the unique person you are.

Natarajasana

The Lord of the Dance or Dancer's Pose

The Sanskrit word *nata* means "dancer" and *raja*, "king". *Nataraja* is one of the names given to the Hindu deity Shiva, referring to him as the cosmic dancer. The dancer's pose is portrayed in many of the statues found in *Nataraja* temples.

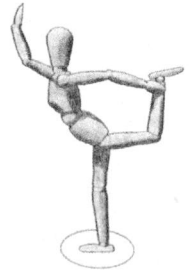

Natarajasana ~ The Lord of the Dance or the Dancer's Pose

In one sense, one might consider a series of postures in yoga to be a dance. By creating unique, graceful, fluid movements linked to the breath you become the choreographer. But in a balance posture, we pause our dance through life to become inquisitive about a single point of focus, the *drishti*, to clear the mind and relax the body.

Uttanasana

Standing Forward Fold

This *asana* is often a component of *Surya namaskar*, the sun salutations. Surya is the Hindu god of the sun and the source of all life who brings light and warmth to the whole world.

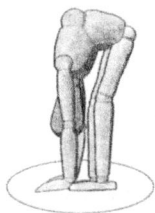

Uttanasana ~ Standing Forward Fold

A wonderful metaphor is the light that exists in each and everyone of us. You possess the power to bring your light and warmth to everyone in your world. One secular translation of *namaste* is "the light within me honors the light within you." May your light become so bright for everyone to see.

Uttanasana is a passive posture. We fold at the hips and let the upper body simply hang. By dangling the arms and shifting the torso ever so slightly, we can experience the force of gravity gently pulling the fingers and arms toward the earth. It is a reminder that there are many forces in nature that go unnoticed, but are dominant in our lives.

Padmasana

The Lotus Pose

The lotus blossom is an important religious symbol in Hinduism and other eastern religions. The Buddha is often depicted in Far Eastern art sitting in the lotus position. In Hinduism, the lotus flower is symbolic of beauty, spirituality and eternity. The lotus flower also represents rebirth as it emerges from muddy and murky waters, transforming into a beautiful, pristine bloom. Yoga is the path to transformation, allowing one's spirit to emerge from the dark, seemingly inescapable place of mental illness into the light of peace and contentment.

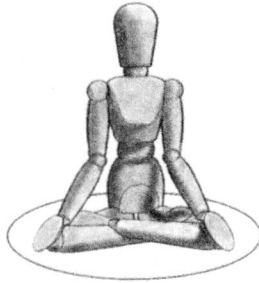

Padmasana ~ The Lotus

Navasana

The Boat Pose or Upward Boat

All of the poses we do have Sanskrit names that are compound words comprised of a root and the word, *asana*, meaning position. "*Nava*" is the Sanskrit root for "boat". Interestingly, in Latin the root for "boat" is "nav". We find this root in English words, such as navy and navigate. Although no direct evidence exists, many linguists believe in the existence of an ancient, common Proto-Indo-European (PIE) language spoken several thousands of years ago, possibly earlier than 4000 BCE, which evolved into known modern languages through diasporas, migrations and interactions of different populations.

Other examples of root similarities are the Sanskrit root for foot "pado" as in the *asana, prasarita padottanasana,* the Greek root "pod" and the Latin root "ped", as in pedal and pedestrian, and the Sanskrit root for knee "janu", as in the *asana, janu shirshasana,* and the Latin

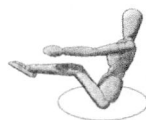

Navasana ~ The Boat Pose

root "genu" as in genuflect. This primordial language would certainly explain the similarity of many of the roots shared between Sanskrit, Greek and the Romance languages. Differences exist between cultures, but ultimately we all share common origins. Although the aforementioned may seem a digression by your author, it illustrates that yoga is more than just a physical practice and, as such, there is a lot of knowledge to be gained and many novel ideas to discover.

Before entering into *navasana,* notice that you are sitting on a triangle formed by the sitz bones and the sacrum/coccyx. Think of that triangle as the keel of your boat that possesses a stabilizing force. The challenge of this posture is to remain sitting on your keel when lifting the feet off of the mat rather than rolling backwards onto the sacrum. This is accomplished twofold: by drawing the thighs into the chest and pulling the chest forward, which thereby shifts weight forward to counteract the backward pull of the upper body as the legs are lifted. In a sense, you are stabilizing your boat whether you are sailing in calm waters or weathering a storm, evening out mood swings and staying afloat despite the difficulties posed by life's challenges.

Virasana
The Hero Pose

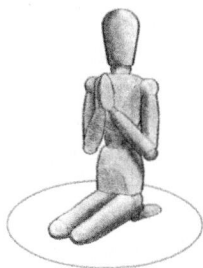

Virasana ~ The Hero's Pose

A hero is typically a courageous, selfless person who achieves greatness, often while effecting change. There is no doubt that to face mental challenges, one must possess courage. In a sense, one enters into a battle with the "monster within" that is depression and anxiety. If the monster is victorious, it will become all-consuming. Yoga stirs up difficult emotions and disturbing thoughts that if faced courageously can neutralize the monster. The monster may never fully retreat from the mind, but its power can be lessened. A change to a positive outlook can ensue, followed by pride in the greatness of your achievement, no matter how large or small it might be. Acceptance is the key to winning the battle, not allowing depression and anxiety to define who you are.

Setu Bandhasana

The Bridge Pose

The bridge pose epitomizes yoga as a personal experience filled with myriad choices to mold your practice to what suits you best, both physically and mentally.

There are many variations available to you in the bridge pose. One might walk the shoulders under the back and interlace fingers. Other options include drawing the arms overhead to either side of the ears, pulling fingertips away from the head, or raising the heels and pressing into the balls of the feet. Both actions can provide greater hip and pelvic elevation with a resultant greater degree of back extension.

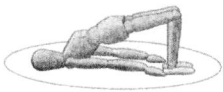

Setu Bandhasana ~ The Bridge Pose

You can breathe life into your bridge by converting a static *asana* into a dynamic, flowing movement. With a deep inhalation, as the pelvis rises, allow the arms to float overhead. With exhalation, the pelvis and arms lower concurrently. The experience can become all your own by adding movements of the fingers and wrists, perhaps not stopping at either end, but rather creating a continuous, graceful flowing motion. By then connecting your breath to the flow, you can become lost in a wonderful moving meditation.

Indudalasana

The Standing Crescent Moon Pose

The *ida nadi* is complementary to the *pingala nadi*, sometimes referred to as the moon and sun energy channels, respectively.

A crescent moon is either waxing or waning. Perhaps, it is waning toward the energy of the sun or waxing toward the full energy of the moon. Either way, while in the crescent moon, we are experiencing a combination of both opposite, yet complimentary energies of the sun and the moon. We create energy and an active body with an outstretched arm and feet grounded firmly into the earth as we activate the energy of the sun. At the same time, as we sustain the pose,

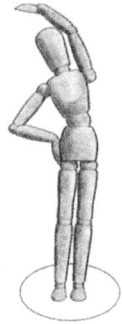

Indudalasana ~ The Standing Crescent Moon Pose

we are afforded time for insight, assessing how we feel and digesting the full experience of your crescent moon.

Salamba Bhujangasana

The Sphinx Pose

In his play *Oedipus Rex,* Sophocles describes the Sphinx, a creature that guarded the city of Thebes, killing those that could not solve her riddle: "What creature walks on four legs in the morning, two legs in the afternoon and three in the evening?" By solving the riddle, Oedipus becomes the King of Thebes and the Sphinx consequently kills herself. His answer describes the life cycle of man, who crawls on four limbs as an infant in the morning of life, walks on two legs as an adult in the afternoon, and walks on three legs in the evening as an elder with a cane.

The riddle is rooted in ancient lore, reflecting the mythology of ancient cultures. Life poses many riddles, many lying in the depths of mystery and yet to be solved. On a personal level, we all are presented with a riddle that each one of us needs to solve in order to determine who we are and why we are here.

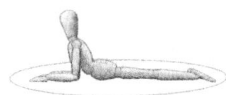

Salamba Bhujangasana ~ The Sphinx Pose

As an *asana,* the sphinx pose is one that engages the body, creating a state of tension. It is not meant to be a passive back-bend, but rather a posture imbued with energy. Activation of the body is achieved through grounding. We begin by firmly pushing the tops of the feet into the mat, followed by the thighs and pelvis, experiencing muscle contraction from feet to hips. We then firmly root into the elbows, forearms and hands to actively raise the chest and intensify the degree of back extension.

We often experience opposites in our yoga practice. Grounding and energizing the body can be done with deep inhalation. With a slow exhalation, all tension in the body can be released. Perhaps, similar to the bridge, you can settle into a mediative flow from tension to release and back again that is connected to the breath.

Bhujangasana
The Cobra Pose

There are many spiritual meanings of the cobra in numerous cultures, possibly best known through the art of ancient Egypt. In Hinduism, the cobra is symbolic of the power and supreme authority of many gods, such as Shiva, the god of transformation.

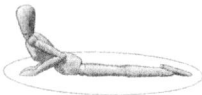

Bhujangasana ~ The Cobra Pose

We might ascribe our own symbolism to the *asana,* such as our innate power that can be accessed to establish mastery of our lives. The cobra possesses the power to kill its prey. Perhaps, we might also consider our cobra to have the power to destroy any negative self-images in the process of personal transformation toward a more positive outlook, imbued with hope for a better future.

Marjaryasana and Bitilasana
The Cat and Cow Poses

The cat and cow poses are complementary poses that are typically done together, flowing from one to the other. The integration of the cat and the cow illustrate pose and counter-pose, one of the important guiding principles of yoga.

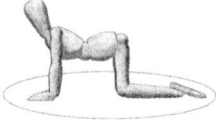

Bitilasana ~ The Cow Pose

These poses afford a wonderful opportunity to experience the connection of the breath to movement and the consequent, ensuing, calming waves of relaxation. In that regard, if you wish, you can assume the table position. Deepen and lengthen your breath. Let the breath begin with the expansion of the belly and like a wave spread up to the collar bones. Then, exhale out all the air that you can. On the next inhalation, as the

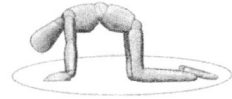

Marjaryasana ~ The Cat Pose

belly expands the tailbone is lifted to the sky. As the breath spreads up into the chest, the sternum is lifted forward, and then the gaze comes up last. Imagine that you are creating two connected waves; the breath that spreads from belly to collar bones and the physical movement that spreads from tailbone to the crown of head. Upon exhalation, the two waves then spread back from the crown of head to the tailbone, as the head first drops, then the back rounds, and finally the tailbone tucks. To take it one step further, imagine that it is the breath that is directing the movement, not the mind. The inhalation opens the body in the cow and the exhalation closes the body in the cat. Single-pointed focus is not on the physical movements or the breath alone, but on the connection of the two.

Closing the eyes can heighten awareness of the other senses. Try an experiment. First, come into your cat and cow with eyes wide open. After several rounds, close your eyes and notice how your experience changes. Are you more aware of the position of your body in space, the sound of deep breathing or the connection of breath to movement?

Salabhasana

The Grasshopper or Locust Pose

As images may be pleasant or disturbing, I prefer to call this *asana* the grasshopper. It is a strenuous pose in which the head, chest, arms and legs are all in the air.

Salabhasana ~ The Grasshopper or Locust Pose

The physicality of this pose presents a wonderful opportunity to engage the power of the mind to divert one's attention away from any straining in the physical body. This is done by creating a single point of focus that clears the mind of other thoughts, including muscle fatigue. One possibility is to create a *drishti* on the front edge of the mat on which to gaze and observe. All thought is devoted to appreciating the qualities of the *drishti,* such as the appearance of the edge of the mat as it differs from the adjacent floor. Another possibility is to focus on the breath. Breathing can be hindered while being supported by the belly, but establishing a deep breath creates a gentle upward and downward pulsation of the body with inhalation and exhalation. The inhalation causes the body to slightly rise as you push your belly into the mat. The exhalation will then result in a slight lowering of the body. Connecting the breath to these subtle movements can be quite meditative. By diverting the mind away from muscular strain to a different point of focus, it can be quite surprising as to how much longer you can sustain this physically challenging pose.

Adho Mukha Svanasana

Downward Dog or Downward Facing Dog

There have been many yoga classes that I have attended where the instructor suggests to relax the body in the downward facing dog pose, implying that this is a comfortable posture. I, for one, have never found that to be the case. I am fine with that. My expectation is that not everything I do in yoga is going to feel good. A similar expectation is a healthy way to go through life. One must accept that life is full of great things and not so great things.

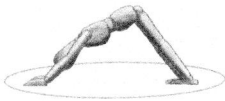

Adho Mukha Svanasana ~ Downward Dog or Downward Facing Dog

To turn discomfort into comfort, numerous options and modifications exist in yoga. In downward facing dog, I can assume a less tense posture by bending the knees with heels off the mat. I can also choose to assume a different, more comfortable posture, such as child's pose, if it enhances my enjoyment and clears my mind of thoughts of discomfort or pain. You should never feel restricted in a yoga class to do what best suits you. In life, except for societal expectations to be a moral person, the only restrictions are self-imposed. A connection to one's true authenticate self can free one from the restrictions on the spirit that result from trying to live up to others' expectations. Life also becomes easier with modifications that create boundaries to steer clear of uncomfortable situations and dysfunctional people.

Urdhva Mukha Svanasana
The Upward Facing Dog

We can easily transition into this pose from the downward facing dog by lowering the pelvis, coming onto and pressing into the tops of the feet, pushing the torso upwards by engaging straight arms and bringing the head and gaze forward.

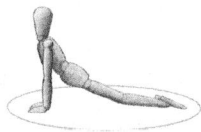

Urdhva Mukha Svanasana ~ The Upward Facing Dog

Perhaps, this transition brings our gaze from an introspective position in downward dog, gazing to what exists behind us, into a forward facing position, looking into the future to consider new possibilities.

Kapotasana

The Pigeon Pose

The Sanskrit word *"kapota"* means pigeon, which has significance in the Hindu religion. Kapoteswara or Kapota Ishwara is one of thousands of names for Shiva, one of the three main Hindu deities. It is written in the ancient text, the *Skanda Purana,* that the Lord Shiva undertook a *tapas,* an ascetic practice performed to achieve purification, that was so severe that living solely on air he shrinks down to the size of a pigeon.

In the full expression of *kapotasana,* the torso is upright, creating a back bend. One might imagine the shape of your body approximating that of a pigeon. A more meditative version of this pose is known as the sleeping

Kapotasana ~ The Pigeon Pose

pigeon, whereby back extension becomes flexion, as the head is brought down to a pillow created by stacked hands or fore-arms. Each long exhalation allows the body to release into the mat.

While in *kapotasana,* one might consider their life struggles as being a *tapas.* As one sinks into the quiet, restful position of *eka pada rajakapotasana,* an opportunity arises to then experience a purification of the mind; eliminating mental clutter and unwanted thoughts.

Eka Pada Rajakapotasana ~The Sleeping Pigeon Pose

Phalakasana
High Plank

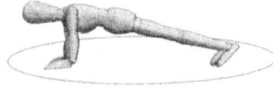

Phalakasana ~ High Plank

Chaturanga Dandasana
Four Limb Staff Pose or Low Pushup

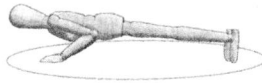

Chaturanga Dandasana ~ Four Limb Staff Pose or Low Pushup

Very often, we progress from high plank to *chaturanga* or low pushup in anticipation of ending in an upward facing dog and then possibly a downward facing dog. When I transition between the two, what I like to focus on are my toes. In the high plank, my toes are curled as I push my heels behind me, creating power and stability, along with my straight, energized arms. As I begin to enter into my low pushup, I roll forward onto the tips of my toes, as my body moves forward and down. Eventually, at the end of the low pushup I will continue the forward motion of my toes to land on the tops of my feet as I prepare to enter into upward dog. Choice abounds in yoga. Sometimes it is nice to focus on something as simple as your toes.

Chakravakasana
The Sunbird

Chakravak is a mythological bird that appears at sunrise, bringing with it warmth and light.

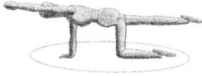

Chakravakasana ~ The Sunbird

The pose is relatively physically challenging, as it requires balancing on one knee and lower leg and the opposite-sided hand and arm. Strength and balance come from grounding into those parts of the body that are on the mat. Once balance is achieved, the process of elongation from toes to fingertips can begin. Imagine two nice friends pulling your fingers and toes in opposite directions. As the stretch ensues, a wonderful line of energy forms that fuels your light and your warmth, as you become the sunbird.

Balasana or Garbhasana

Child's Pose

There are several variations of this *asana*. One common variation brings the feet to touch, knees wide apart, and elbows, forearms and forehead resting on the mat. One can also position the feet and knees together to touch, drawing the arms back next to the feet as the forehead drops to the mat. Whatever expression you choose, it should be a position to decrease muscle tension as much as possible. The forehead must be supported to fully relax the muscles of the neck. The head weighs ten to fifteen pounds. Having the equivalent of a bowling ball floating in the air and pulling on the neck can cloud the mind with muscle tension and be a distraction in this mediative posture.

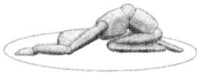

*Balasana or Garbhasana
~ Child's Pose*

If one is unable to relax the forehead on the mat, relaxing the neck muscles can be facilitated by resting the forehead on a block, stacked hands or stacked forearms. Even if you are able to rest the forehead directly on the mat, experiment with making a pillow with stacked hands or forearms to see if you experience a lessening of any neck and shoulder strain you weren't even aware of. In addition, if it is not physically possible to fully bring the sitz bones to rest on the heels, a blanket can be inserted between the two. Any sensations of physical discomfort will interfere with the enjoyment of a time of stillness, rest and relaxation, and one where you can be with yourself and your thoughts.

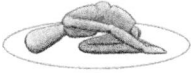

Balasana or Garbhasana ~ Child's Pose Variation

Perhaps, it is the child within us that must be rediscovered or revisited; that time of innocence before our minds were usurped by the stresses of life. An exploration of childhood influences can give insight into one's personality and present relationships. Of course, many of us have childhood traumas. Just as we practice yoga near our physical edge, the point at which discomfort in a pose arises, we must also not move beyond our mental edge by entering into a distressing emotional place.

The *asanas* are an opportunity to position the body in unique ways. The power of each posture to elevate the spirit lies in the individual interpretation and personalization of the experience. Your experience is yours to create. You become the artist by ascribing personal meaning to each pose in the context of life experiences, historical references, the action of the physical body and the engagement of the senses. Each time you practice yoga, another opportunity arises to use your imagination, creativity and intellect to draw your emotions and thoughts into the present moment. Being in that moment is at the heart of learned relaxation. That moment is yours to enjoy!

10

POSTURE SEQUENCES TO DE-STRESS

Posture sequences are any series of *asanas* linked to the breath. Deep inhalations and exhalations direct the body's movements through the transitions between poses. And if sustaining a static pose without movement, continued heightened awareness of the breath remains uninterrupted. Posture sequences can take on a life of their own through a deep profound intention to consider their meanings in the context of one's own life journey.

All of the following posture sequences will be more effective in reducing stress if the breath is first established in stillness before the body begins to move. To that end, we turn to *pranayama*, the yogic breathing techniques; discussed in a later chapter on breathing into relaxation. We start with the foundational breath for the practice of *pranayama, dirga pranayama,* or the complete breath. Let the breath slowly evolve from your normal breathing rhythm to deep, slow diaphragmatic breaths. As you will see later on, *dirga pranayama* is a three part breath. At first, be deliberate about incorporating the three parts of *dirga* breathing: the belly, ribs and upper chest. Once you are inhaling into complete fullness and exhaling into complete emptiness, allow the three parts to become one. Imagine a wave moving toward the shore as the breath proceeds from the belly up to the chest, and then the wave returning back out to sea as you exhale out all the air you can. Layering on the another type of *pranayama*, the *ujjayi* breath, which is created with a small constriction in the back of the throat, reinforces the image of the shore, with the sound of the waves amplified by your inhalations and exhalations. You might also consider a few rounds of alternate nostril breathing, or *nadi shodhana,* to further clear the energy channels before entering into a posture sequence, allowing for the calming flow of relaxation to more easily spread throughout all parts of the body and mind.

Once the breath is established and you are centered in the present moment, you may then enter into any of the posture sequences that follow or one that is your own creation. In a yoga class, the sequence of postures are chosen by the instructor for his, her or their students. In the process of learned relaxation and in your own practice, you are the both the teacher and student and you have an opportunity to write your own curriculum.

Setting aside time for self care should be a priority. In this hectic world, it is often difficult to carve out time from a busy schedule. Many possess the notion that yoga must be done for an hour or so in a class. I have heard innumerable times from people living busy lives that there is not enough time in the day for yoga; getting to a class just doesn't fit into their schedules. The truth is that you can establish your own regular practice at home by using any of the following posture sequences and/or your own creations in conjunction with establishing the breath and warming up the body. In addition, seemingly limitless online videos of varying lengths are more time efficient than attending a class in a studio or other venue. Ultimately, by making yoga a part of your day, improved concentration and focus will increase productivity and actually create more time for self-care.

Yoga can be done for any amount of time. Arguably, a practice done at home daily for fifteen or twenty minutes is much more effective for stress reduction and promoting well-being than a practice done in a class a couple of times a week. Once established as a routine, that short daily practice can become your sanctuary, a safe space away from the pressures of life. After a while, possibly over several weeks, yoga becomes part of your daily routine as the brain learns feelings of relaxation triggered by simple movements linked to deep breathing. Those feelings elicited by a short daily practice can be accessed at any time during a hectic day. When something isn't going your way, immediate stress reduction may be as easy as a single sun breath with movement linked to a deep diaphragmatic inhalation and a complete slow exhalation. Doing a mini yoga routine at any time during the day resets the brain and lessens stress and anxiety.

Yoga teaches us that we have choice. If you wish to create your own posture sequence, you can choose the specific *asanas* to perform and, more importantly, which postures are most comfortable for you. Of course, don't have the expectation that everything in yoga is supposed to feel good. In my own practice, I try to listen to the needs of my body in identifying which *asana* speaks to me at any given moment.

I would love to tell you that there are a specific series of *asanas* that promote relaxation more than others. The following themed posture sequences are my own creations. I believe that their power to relax lies in the presentation of novel ideas that can serve as a focus for your practice. Regardless of which *asanas* comprise a posture sequence, it will have the power to relax if you experience it in the present moment. A posture sequence should also include periods of stillness in which to digest the experience. It bears repeating, "The magic of yoga lies in the spaces between the postures." Always have an awareness of the breath and afford yourself time for reflection.

How do we progress through a posture sequence? Quite simply, we sustain an *asana* for a variable amount of time until we transition into another. The movements of the body for each transition are connected to the breath by inhaling a part of the anatomy to a particular position in space and exhaling it to another.

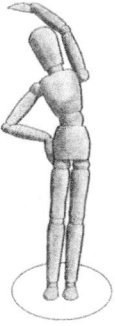

For example, starting in *tadasana,* one might inhale an arm directly overhead and then exhale it over to the opposite side of the body to enter into *indudalasana,* the standing crescent moon pose. A subsequent inhalation may bring the arm back up overhead and the torso back to center, and the next exhalation back into *indudalasana.*

Indudalasana ~ The Standing Crescent Moon Pose

Repeating these movements that are directed by the breath creates a flowing motion. By flexing and extending the wrist, the movement can become more graceful. If imbalance is not an issue, the eyes can be closed to better sink into the meditative effects of this breath-directed flow of movement.

In yoga, we strive to connect the inhalation to movements that open up the body, especially the chest and belly, and the exhalation to those that close down the body. One example is a sun breath. With inhalation the arms are swept overhead as the body lengthens and the chest opens up towards the sky with a gentle back bend. The exhalation initiates a swan dive down to *uttanasana,* or the standing forward fold. From a practical standpoint, this makes perfect sense. Sweeping the arms overhead and lengthening the torso with a straight spine allows more room for the downward excursion of the diaphragm into the belly to produce a deeper inhalation. Folding forward crunches the abdomen, which helps to expel air out of the lungs with exhalation. From a spiritual perspective, the deep inhalation of *prana* opens up the body, allowing for greater receptivity of the positive energy of the life force. Closing down the body with exhalation better rids the body of mental waste and negative energy.

Rather than breathing into movements to create transitions, one can also breathe into a stretch while sustaining a static posture. In the above example of *indulasana*, the crescent-shaped stretch that develops in the side body is a wonderful target for a deep inhalation. One can also breathe into a *drishti*, a visual focal point; imagining the point

Uttanasana ~ Standing Forward Fold

being drawn closer and closer to the eyes with each breath. And although it may not be self-evident, you can also breathe into a thought, idea or emotion that appears on the blank slate of mental clarity.

Before practicing any specific posture sequences or performing any activity, it is paramount to warmup the body to increase its efficiency and prevent injury. At one point in my life, I ran a few miles on a daily basis. Before setting off on a run, my warmup consisted of a couple of quick stretches of both legs and then I was off. Aside from being at a greater risk for injury, I didn't understand that if I had done a more thor-

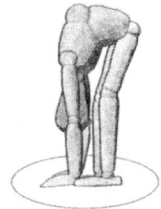

ough warmup of my body, I would have been able to run more efficiently, likely with a faster pace and for longer periods of time before tiring. Before any physical activity, including sustaining any of the *asanas,* it is critical to progressively and gradually move joints, stretch muscles and loosen up the spine.

Warming up joints consists of lubricating them and stretching the relatively stiff connective tissues that comprise the joint, including the joint capsule, associated ligaments and fascia. Moving and opening the joints spreads synovial fluid throughout, allowing for smooth gliding of one surface over another. It is analogous to motor oil lubricating the pistons of an engine. As the engine warms up, oil is spread evenly over the surfaces of the pistons, assuring smooth motion, while at the same time preventing wear and tear.

Muscles must be progressively stretched to prevent micro tears and establish adequate blood flow and oxygenation. Increasing the heart rate also increases the delivery of nutrients and oxygen to the muscles. Returning back to the car analogy, if time is taken to prime the engine, it will operate more efficiently.

I approach warming up the spine as if it is an isolated entity, although in actuality, along with the bones, it is also comprised of joints and associated muscles. The spine is capable of moving in six directions. Since the spine is involved in all of the *asanas,* warm-ups should always include these six motions:

- flexion, or bending forward
- extension, or arching back
- lateral flexion, or bending side to side to the right and left
- twisting to the right and left

Warmups are necessary before any activity is initiated, but they are also a wonderful way to start the day. Upon awakening, a fifteen minute warmup routine energizes mind and body, setting a healthy tone before taking on the challenges of work or the daily care of home or family.

In yoga, a specific technique of standing warmups is called *dasha chalana,* or the eight churnings, which are eight specific movements of the joints and spine. Traditionally, *dasha chalana* consists of ankle rotations, knee circles, hip circles, shoulder rolls, spinal twists, spinal waves, neck circles and wrist circles. I add additional movements to assure that the entire body is ready for any physical activity. As long as you are warming up all of the joints, muscles and the spine, any series of movements you choose will be effective.

To practice a relatively straightforward warmup routine, find a chair or come to stand. Elongate the spine and relax the shoulders. Start with several deep belly breaths. Imagine inhaling in positive energy. Let the exhalations relax, gently pulling the entire body towards the ground and the shoulder blades down the back. Once a deep breath is established, proceed to warming up the body.

An easy method to warmup the joints consists of progressing from the ground up:

- wiggling and spreading the toes
- circling the ankles
- flexing and extending the knees
- circling the hips
- rotating the shoulders
- flexing and extending the elbows
- circling the wrists
- moving the joints of the hand and fingers

Similarly, we can warmup the muscles from ground up:

- flexing and extending the toes to warm up the intrinsic muscles of the foot
- flexing, extending and circling the ankles to warm up the muscles of the calf
- with a flat back, hinging forward at the hips creases with a straightened leg to stretch the hamstrings, or in a chair, raising a straight leg and alternating between pointing the toes and pushing out through the heel
- grabbing a bent knee to the chest to stretch the quadriceps muscles
- spreading legs wide to stretch the hip adductors, or inner thigh muscles

- alternating flexing and extending the elbow to stretch the triceps and biceps muscles, respectively
- flexing, extending and circling the wrists to stretch the muscles of the forearm
- spreading fingers wide and making a fist to stretch and contract the intrinsic muscles of the hand

Finally, we move the spine in its six directions:

- alternating arching and rounding the back
- sweeping an arm over the head to bend to the side for lateral flexion and then repeating on the other side
- twisting from side to side

Taking fifteen with the aforementioned routine is a wonderful way to start your day. Once the body is warmed up, it is time to either engage the mind with self-reflection to ease into what lies ahead for your day or you can extend your practice by proceeding to a posture sequence.

I have entitled the following posture sequences to emphasize their meaning, intention and symbolism, with the hope of stimulating thought and a mind that is active in the present moment. Each one embodies different qualities of the human condition. One sequence may resonate with you more than others. The majority of the *asanas* presented are illustrated in the preceding chapter. In addition, as you consider these sequences, remember a major proviso in this book, "Don't do anything that is uncomfortable, either mentally or physically."

Considering posture sequences as musical passages that delight the spirit, make sure to insert rests or pauses in order to breathe and reflect. As you reflect on your experience, practice non-attachment and don't have any expectations. It is fine if you have life-changing revelations or you think nothing particularly remarkable has happened. At the very least, taking a pause with a deep breath will rest the physical body, allow muscles to recover and induce physiological-mediated relaxation. Non-attachment allows you to enjoy the moment rather than be distracted by the implications of success or failure. As you practice, always honor the mind and body with kindness. Beyond the personal meaning that any of these posture sequences may possess, let it be gratitude for yourself, your loved ones and all of life's blessings that energize your mind and body.

As much as I stress relaxation through your yoga practice, enjoyment is arguably equally important. So, please enjoy the following eight posture sequences:

- **The Warrior**
- **Lines of Energy**
- **The Child**
- **Novelty and Living in the Moment**
- **Honoring the Spine**
- **Less is More**
- **Creating Balance**
- **Feet First**
- **The Posture Sequence of Self-Kindness**

THE WARRIOR

- *Tadasana ~ The Mountain*
- *Utthita tadasana ~ The Star*
- *Virabhadrasana II ~ Warrior II*
- *Viparita virabhadrasana ~ The Reverse Warrior*
- *Utthita parsvakonasana ~ The Extended Angle*
- *Tasdasana ~ The Mountain*
- *Stillness with Hands in Anjali Mudra at Heart Center*
- *Virabhadrasana I ~ Warrior I*
- *Baddha virabhadrasana ~ The Humble Warrior*

- *Tadasana ~ The Mountain*
- *Stillness with Hands in Anjali Mudra at Heart Center*

This sequence is about tapping into the strength of the warrior, both physically and mentally. You might reflect on how you might be a warrior in life, with pride in any attempt to take on life's challenges. Unfortunately for many, however, dealing with mental disease can be a lifelong battle and being the warrior requires courage and the drive to fight for peace and contentment.

1. Facing the long edge of your mat, begin in **tadasana,** the mountain pose. *Tadasana* is our first opportunity to harness the power of our inner warrior. Like a mountain with a large base of attachment on the earth, we actively ground our feet into the mat, followed by an upward, activating flow of energy, as the body stretches skyward like the tall summit of our mountain.

2. From *tadasana,* widen your stance, feet about a leg length apart and parallel or slightly pigeon-toed.

3. Raise arms up to shoulder height to come into **utthita tadasana**, the star pose. While continuing to ground both feet into the mat, pull fingers in opposite directions to maximize the stretch in the arms. Three lines of energy will develop, two arising from the earth, spreading up both legs, and one

extending through straight, outstretched arms. The lines of energy intersect at the heart *chakra,* the energy center for love and compassion, the qualities of a benevolent warrior.

4. From *utthita tadasana,* we can easily transition into **virabhadrasana II**, warrior II. Continuing to engage the arms and legs, rotate one foot ninety degrees, such that the front foot and back foot are aligned and perpendicular. Palms are both face down. Rotate the head ninety degrees to look out beyond the front hand, possibly focusing on challenges that lie ahead or new possibilities on the horizon. Both the rotation of the foot and head should be isolated movements; the rest of the body remaining motionless. Finally, keeping shoulders over hips, slowly bend the front knee, translating it forward over the front ankle. Do a quick body scan: feet perpendicular in a single line, leg muscles engaged, knee over front ankle, chest rotated to face the long edge of the mat, arms actively stretched and parallel, shoulders over hips, and gaze out over front hand. While sustaining *virabhadrasana,* become aware of a deep breath. Imagine the breath spreading down the legs and out through the arms. Enjoy a newfound strength and always remember that you have the power to create that strength. It comes from within. It is

under your control. Embrace the strength of your warrior.

5. Now, rotate the front palm to face the ceiling. With the next deep inhalation, sweep the front palm up and overhead, transitioning into ***viparita virabhadrasana***, the reverse warrior. Extend the fingers toward the back wall as you pull the upper shoulder up and behind you to open up the chest to the sky, coming into a spiritually receptive posture.

6. Take a deep breath. On a slow exhalation, slowly windmill the arms forward, bringing the forearm of the front arm on to the thigh of the front leg, sweeping the back arm up and forward, to come into ***utthita parsvakonasana***, the extended angle pose. Align the overhead, straight arm with the extended back leg to create a single straight, diagonal line that becomes a conduit through which energy flows from earth to sky.

7. Return back to warrior II, rotate the chest ninety degrees to face the front of the mat, shift weight forward, step the back leg forward to meet the front, and return to ***tadasana***. Sweep your arms overhead with a deep inhalation, palms coming together in ***anjali mudra***, or prayer hands. With a slow exhalation, release all tension in the body as the palms drift down to heart center. Come into stillness. Now, it is your time to digest the

experience. You might notice physical sensations. Maybe one side of the body feels different than the other. Or allow thoughts and emotions to arise without expectations of achieving any insight. Stay in stillness as long as you wish. We rush through life so often. It is wonderful to take time to be aware and mindful.

8. Once you are ready to reactivate the physical body, step to the back of your mat, chest facing toward the front edge. Position the feet wider than you would for the mountain, about twelve inches apart. With hands on hips, take a large step directly forward, as if you are stepping through a door into a brand new space, a place of strength and wisdom. The shoulders, chest, and hips should all remain facing forward toward the front edge of the mat. Rotate the back foot forty-five degrees. Bend the front knee over the front ankle. Sweep the arms into a vee-shape to enter into *virabhadrasana I*, the warrior I. "Vee" is for victory as we become the warrior.

9. Let the palms meet overhead. With a slow exhalation, bring the hands together in *anjali mudra* at heart center. Hinge forward at the hip creases with a flat back to come into *baddha virabhadrasana*, the humble warrior. Humility is not the act of denigrating or underestimating one's abilities, but rather an acceptance of yourself as you are. You can

be a more successful warrior in life with the realization that the only limitation to personal growth is thinking that you have any limitations. In yoga, the possibilities for touching the spirit are limitless.

10. Bring the hands to the hips, shift weight forward and step to the front of the mat, returning back to *tadasana.* Sweep the arms overhead and slowly let the hands in **anjali mudra** return to heart center. Return to stillness. Some feel that the energy of the heart *chakra* exits through the palms. With the palms connected at heart center, a positive feedback loop is created with the energy of love, compassion and gratitude exiting and re-entering the body, growing in magnitude with each revolution. Enjoy that energy, possibly creating an image in the mind of someone or something for which you are grateful. Breathe deeply into feelings of gratitude. Gratitude leads to all of the other positive emotions we experience, including the pride and heightened self-esteem of your warrior.

11. Now, as you repeat this posture sequence on the other side, notice if the experience changes. Does one side of the body feel differently than the other? Are different thoughts and emotions arising? Once again, it is important to practice non-attachment in yoga, approaching it with no expectations. Maybe

something will speak to you and change your perspective, or maybe nothing mentally engaging will happen. Either result is fine. Simply, enjoy the process. Most importantly, a warrior should be proud of any attempt to overcome challenges, whether successful or not. Be the warrior! Be proud!

LINES OF ENERGY

- *Tadasana ~ The Mountain*
- *Indudalasana ~ Standing Half Crescent Moon Pose*
- *Utthita Tadasana ~ The Star*
- *Virabhadrasana II ~ Warrior II*
- *Utthita Parsvakonasana ~ The Extended Angle*
- *Viparita Trikonasana ~ Reverse Triangle Pose*
- *Utthita Tadasana ~ The Star*
- *Virabhadrasana II ~ Warrior II*
- *Utthita Parsvakonasana ~ The Extended Angle*
- *Viparita Trikonasana ~ Reverse Triangle Pose*
- *Phalakasana ~ High Plank*
- *Chakravakasana ~ The Sunbird*
- *Balasana ~ Child's Pose*

As an exercise, close your eyes and take a moment to bring your arms to shoulder height. Notice that you have created a straight line from finger tip to finger tip. Now stretch the arms in opposite directions as if two good friends are gently pulling on your hands. The stretch activates and engages your arm muscles, as well as the muscles of the chest and shoulders, thereby creating a line of energy from fingertip to fingertip.

Creating your own unique experience in your yoga practice, and ultimately in life, comes from the ability to generate inner energy using the imagination coupled with an active physical body. Depression and anxiety can deplete energy, making it difficult to muster the strength to practice self-care. Imagining lines of energy in your yoga practice can teach you how to better energize the mind in order to be better positioned to take positive action.

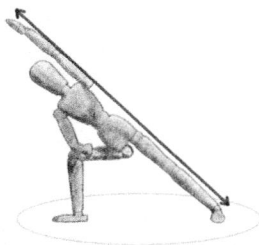

Utthita Parsvakonasana ~ Extended Side Angle Pose and the line of energy that connects earth to sky

Return to the above exercise and recreate the line of energy from fingertip to fingertip. Breathe deeply into that line, its power growing exponentially with each breath. Imagine the energy flooding the body and spirit. With your next exhalation, relax your arms as if your two good friends let go and observe the feeling of relaxation that spreads throughout the arms and chest. In yoga, it is the interplay between engagement and relaxation that gives us a greater appreciation for both than if experienced separately. With your next inhalation, stretch out your arms as the energy returns. Relax with your next exhalation. Alternating between the two states of activation and rest coupled with your inhalations and exhalations teaches the mind to both harness and release energy; to both engage and relax. As you move through this posture sequence, use the breath to inhale in positive energy and exhale into relaxation.

At the heart of learned relaxation is learning to be in the moment and releasing thoughts that don't serve in the present. Lines of energy are useful constructs that serve as another source of single-pointed focus. Always keep in mind, you are the one that possesses and controls the power to attribute positive energy to the physical lines you assume. The energy you experience arises from two sources. One is the heat that emanates from active muscles. The other comes from creative thoughts arising from an active imagination. Enjoy the energy and images that you create.

1. Begin in *tadasana*, the mountain pose. Sweep the arms overhead. Inhale deeply into two forces, one from the grounding of the feet into the mat, the other from stretching the arms upwards by pulling

fingertips toward the ceiling. Those opposing forces energize the entire body, as a line of energy forms that extends from the feet to the fingertips, connecting earth to sky. On your next exhalation, release all of the energy as if you took a piece of taut yarn and let it loosely fall to the ground. Breathe into relaxation. On your next inhalation, activate the body to re-create your line of energy and enjoy a full body stretch.

2. Grab one wrist, say the right, with the opposite hand and actively pull the right arm straight up towards the sky, once again forming a vertical line of energy. Maintaining length in the body, use your left arm strength to pull the right wrist over to the left. Consequently, the body will arch to the left. Imagine that you are bending the straight, vertical line of energy from *tadasana* into a long arc that extends along the side body in **indudalasana**, the standing half crescent moon pose. Switch hands, grabbing the left wrist with the right hand, and bend your line of energy to the opposite side. Breathe deeply into the wonderful stretch along the side body. Feel the energy grow with each inhalation. Once again, release and relax into your exhalation.

3. Come back to center, and with a long exhalation allow the arms to slowly descend. Turn ninety

degrees on your mat. With hands on the hips, take a large step apart with the feet, about a leg length apart if possible, feet are parallel or slightly pigeon-toed. Bring the arms up to an approximate forty-five degree angle to become the star, **utthita tadasana.** Actively ground feet into the mat and pull fingertips away from the body to energize your star. Experience four diagonal lines of energy; two radiating up both arms and two down both legs, all originating from the heart *chakra,* the energy center for love, compassion and gratitude. Like a beautiful, twinkling star, you are emitting your warmth into the universe.

4. To transition into **virabhadrasana II**, warrior II, lower the arms to the level of the shoulders, rotate one foot and your gaze ninety degrees and bend your front knee over the ankle. Once again, you possess the power to energize the body. Identify the lines of energy that form by activating the arms and legs. For a few deep breaths become the powerful warrior.

5. When you are ready, with a long exhalation, drop your front forearm onto your front thigh and bring your back arm overhead at about a forty-five degree angle to enter into the full expression of **utthita parsvakonasana**, the extended angle pose. The arm overhead forms a diagonal line with the extended

back leg. Ground the back foot into the mat and pull fingers of the overhead arm in the opposite direction and inhale deeply into a line of energy that connects the earth to your place above in the infinite universe.

6. Return back to warrior II. Straighten your front leg. Keeping the arms level, like the hands on a clockface, rotate them back into a diagonal line to enter into *viparita trikonasana*, the reverse triangle pose. Pull fingertips in opposite directions to energize the arms. As you gaze over the fingertips reaching up, imagine energy shooting out into the sky or being set to launch a ball of energy with a sling shot up into the air. Additional lines of energy extend down both legs into the earth below.

7. Return back to the star pose and repeat steps 4-6 on the other side. Experiencing the same poses on the other side of the body is an opportunity to witness the asymmetry that exists in our seemingly symmetric bodies.

8. After you have completed step 6 on the other side of your body, with exhalation, bend the front knee and windmill the arms forward in order to frame the front foot with both hands on the mat. Step back into *phalakasana*, high plank. Strength and balance come from pressing hands into the mat and pushing heels back, grounding into the balls of the

feet. Once again, breathe deeply into the line of energy that forms throughout a straight, supported body.

9. Drop both knees directly under the hips and transition into table position. Lift one leg and the opposite-sided arm parallel to the ground to come into *chakravakasana*, the sunbird. Allow the line of energy to develop from fingertips to toes by stretching the arm and leg to lengthen the entire body. Imagine those two good friends returning to gently pull your hand and foot in opposite directions. Repeat with the opposite arm and leg.

10. Return to table. Then push back into *balasana*, child's pose. It is now time to come into stillness and reflect on your experience. Release any tension from the body. Allow any residual energy that surged through the lines in your body that you created to dissipate and fade away. Make sure the forehead is supported by the mat, stacked hands, forearms, or fists, or a yoga block to soften the shoulders and neck. Stay right here for as long as you wish. Simply enjoy the moment, a moment of peace.

THE CHILD

- *Tadasana ~ The Mountain*
- *Uttanasana ~ Standing Forward Fold*
- *Phalakasana ~ High Plank*
- *Chaturanga Dandasana ~ Low Pushup*
- *Urdhva Mukha Svanasana ~ Upward Facing Dog*
- *Adho Mukha Svanasana ~ Downward Facing Dog*
- *Balasana ~ Child's Pose*
- *Bharmasana ~ Table Pose*
- *Chakravakasana ~ The Sunbird*
- *Salabhasana ~ The Grasshopper*
- *Balasana ~ Child's Pose*
- *Bharmasana ~ Table Pose*
- *Adho Mukha Svanasana ~ Downward Facing Dog*
- *Urdhva Mukha Svanasana ~ Upward Facing Dog*
- *Reverse Chaturanga Dandasana ~ High Pushup*
- *Phalakasana ~ High Plank*
- *Adho Mukha Svanasana ~ Downward Facing Dog*
- *Balasana ~ Child's Pose*

Throughout the course of a day, a child is very active, but at the same time requires periods of rest. We try to create a balance in our yoga practice; a balance of mind and body, activity and rest, and mindfulness of the external world with insight and introspection. This posture sequence attempts to do just that by interspersing the solitude and stillness of child's pose, or *balasana,* with more active and vigorous poses. By entering into the stillness of the child's pose, an opportunity arises to digest the active physical experience, witness emotions and feelings, direct awareness inward and simply relax.

In child's pose, losing full awareness of the physical body by eliminating any muscular tension is paramount. Any physical discomfort will cloud the mind, obscuring what lies within. To that end, and as mentioned in the previous chapter, it is critical to support the forehead. The head weighs on order of ten to fifteen pounds, and allowing it to dangle in space creates undue tension on the neck and shoulders. While in child's pose, if the forehead does not reach the mat, support it with stacked hands, forearms, stacked fists or a yoga block. Even if the forehead does reach the mat, try creating a pillow for the forehead with stacked hands to see if any residual tension in the neck and shoulders, of which you were unaware, disappears. In addition, if your hips do not touch your heels, you might consider placing a rolled blanket between the two.

Many of the *asanas* of this posture sequence are found in a typical *vinyasa* flow class, which is often relatively fast-paced. A slower approach allows for more time to appreciate the actions of the physical body and the connection of the breath to your movements, with an arguably greater potential for inducing relaxation and states of inwardness. Feel free to linger in any of the *asanas* with the intention of self-inquiry.

Once again, it seems we are always rushing through life. Take your time and enjoy the moment.

1. Begin in **tadasana**, the mountain pose, facing the front of the mat. Once again, become aware of the energy you create through the act of grounding, forming a single line of energy surging through the body, connecting earth to sky.

2. Cross your forearms in front of your belly. While continuing to ground the feet into the mat, inhale the arms overhead, stretching out the arms in opposite directions by pulling fingers away from the body. This sun breath causes warmth to radiate from the center of your body outward and fuels the *agni*, your inner fire.

3. Pause for a long breath to enjoy a full body stretch before swan-diving down into **uttanasana**, the standing forward fold. This *asana* is a passive one. Folding occurs at the hips, as the upper body passively hangs in space. Experiment with letting the hands dangle as you make micro-movements with the torso, allowing gravity to gently pull the arms downward and gain awareness of a force of nature of which we are typically unaware. *Uttanasana* is the act of folding into relaxation.

4. Now, plant your hands on the mat and step one foot back and then other, entering into **phalakasana**, the

high plank. Strength and stability come from firmly pressing hands into the mat and actively pushing heels away from the body. Sustain the high plank as long as it remains comfortable. Focus on deep diaphragmatic breathing.

5. Come onto the tips of the toes and, while maintaining a flat body, lower down into *chatturanga dandasana*, the low pushup. To instill more vigor into the posture, you can allow the body to hover just above the mat for a breath or two. As always, however, practice at your edge to prevent discomfort and potential injury. To that end, in order to lessen stress on the shoulders, arms and wrists, feel free to first drop the knees to the mat before lowering the upper body.

6. Bring the tops of the feet to rest on the mat. Press into the hands to lift the torso and hips into *urdhva mukha svanasana*, upward facing dog. Increase back extension by firmly pressing into the hands and passively dropping the hips, imagining them to be the bottom of a sagging hammock. Once again, to instill more vigor into the posture, consider the option of pressing the tops of the feet into the mat to lift the knees while in upward facing dog, remembering that options are not challenges, but different ways to experience your yoga. Yoga is not a competitive sport.

7. Curl the toes and push back into **adho mukha svanasana**, downward facing dog. Take a few moments to experiment with movement; maybe pedaling the feet or swaying the hips side to side.

8. Drop the knees and settle back into **balasana**, the child's pose. Relax the physical body and divert attention to your thoughts, or at the very least, enjoy a respite from the physicality of this posture sequence. Relax in child's pose for as long as you wish.

9. Without a rush, when you are ready, slide forward into **bharmasana,** the table pose.

10. Extend one leg back at hip height and the opposite sided arm forward at should height, entering into **chakravakasana**, the sunbird. Stability and strength arise from actively grounding the opposite hand and lower leg into the mat. Repeat on the opposite side. Sunbirds are brightly colored birds that feed on nectar. Connect with your inner sunbird and enjoy the sweetness of life.

11. After returning back to table position, lower the body to lie prone on your mat, palms face down at the sides and face resting on chin or forehead. Inhale chest, arms and legs up off the mat to enter into **salabhasana**, the grasshopper pose. To prevent neck strain, do not bend the neck. Rather, let your gaze be directed downward onto the front edge of

your mat to maintain straight alignment of the cervical and thoracic spines. Stay in this posture for as short or long as you wish. Often, when we sustain strenuous postures in yoga we lose awareness of the breath. Maintaining and drawing your focus to deep breathing will allow you to sustain the posture for longer periods of time, drawing thoughts away from any straining in the body. Another way to enjoy *salabhasana* is to convert a static position to a dynamic one, letting the arms and legs pulsate every so slightly up and down with the breath, injecting living energy into your grasshopper.

12. From *salabhasana,* push back once again into **balasana.** The heat and energy of the grasshopper becomes the relaxing stillness of the child. In yoga, as in life, we often encounter opposite sensations that give us a greater appreciation for each one than if both were experienced separately. A frigid day gains new meaning when stepping into a warm and toasty house. Once again, remain in the child's pose for as long as you wish. It is once again time to relax the body and connect with the mind.

13. When ready, you may slide forward back into table position, curl the toes and push back into downward facing dog. Bring your gaze forward between your hands and walk your feet forward,

returning to the standing forward fold. Cross your forearms. With your next inhalation, sweep the arms up overhead as your torso rises back into an upright position with a big sun breath. Let the palms touch overhead. With your next slow exhalation, allow the palms to drift down to heart center and come into stillness, one of greater receptivity to any new ideas or perspectives arising from this energetically balanced posture sequence.

14. Option to repeat the posture sequence, possibly increasing the pace of transitions between *asanas* to see how it changes your experience. Experimentation keeps your yoga fresh and interesting.

NOVELTY AND LIVING IN THE MOMENT

- *Tadasana ~ The Mountain*
- *Utthita Hasta Padangusthasana Variation ~ Standing Crane Pose*
- *Utthita Tadasana ~ The Star*
- *Utkata Konasana ~ The Goddess Pose*
- *Virabhadrasana II ~ Warrior II*
- *Viparita virabhadrasana ~ The Reverse Warrior*
- *Utthita parsvakonasana ~ The Extended Angle*

- *Prasarita padottanasana ~ Wide Angle Standing Forward Fold*
- *Adho Mukha Svanasana ~ Downward Facing Dog*

This following scenario may resonate with you. When I drive my car home from work, I take the same route each day. The route has become so familiar that without the need to concentrate on where I'm going, my mind has a chance to wander to thoughts about anything and everything except about what is happening in front of me at that moment. In fact, I can become so engrossed in my thoughts that after a time I often experience a sought of re-awakening that brings my conscious attention back to the road with a frightening realization that for some time I didn't actually remember driving my car. My mind was on autopilot. I was physically driving my car in the present moment, but due to the familiarity of my experience, my thoughts were on everything other than what was occurring in that moment.

Learned relaxation requires mindfulness of the moment. Often, we repeat habitual behaviors without conscious, directed thought. In fact, the greater the familiarity of whatever you may be doing, the more opportunity there is for the mind to wander elsewhere. Such can be true in the practice of yoga. A teacher might tell you to come into a warrior II pose. If you have been practicing yoga for a while, you might just pop right into the pose. In fact, through muscle memory, you assume the pose the same exact way every time. There is no need to focus on the position of the arms, legs and torso. They are where they need to be for your own expression of the pose. Without the need to focus on what is happening in the body, the mind can go elsewhere; anywhere from lamentations on the past to worries about the future, or even the need to remember to pick up milk on the way home. When what we do or think becomes habitual and familiar, novelty is required to redirect the mind back into the present moment. Driving home from work by a new route or putting on your pants with the opposite leg first requires much more concentration than doing those things in a familiar, habitual manner.

You can try an experiment. Assume a yoga posture. For example, come into warrior I as you typically do. With the arms overhead, simply bring the palms together to touch. Conscious thought is required to move the arms so that the palms can come together, followed by conscious awareness of the new sensation of the touch of the hands. Even though the brain sends and receives millions of signals every second, we can only focus on one thought at a time. Even when experiencing a cacophony of mind chatter, ultimately we only consider one thought at a time, even if those thoughts are racing out of control. Since you only have the capacity for experiencing a single thought at any given moment, it is impossible not to bring your full awareness to the movement of your arms or the touch of your palms. Even if it is only for a short time, you are focusing and thinking in the moment. Your palms are touching in the present, eliciting a single thought, the only one of which you are aware at the time.

The introduction of novelty into your yoga practice is another way to achieve mindfulness. In addition, *asanas* need not be static. We typically sustain postures in a single position, but the introduction of movement or flow transforms the familiar static poses into dynamic ones. While in a flow of movement, the body assumes new positions and configurations that, with deliberate focus, can activate the mind with novel thoughts that can be emotionally impactful. That flow can also be connected to the breath to facilitate feelings of inwardness, mental clarity and relaxation.

I have taught yoga for five years at the time of writing this book and practiced yoga for close to six. During my initial yoga teacher training at the Kripalu Center for Yoga and Health, I learned how to guide students through twenty-one traditional *asanas*. I have added several more to my repertoire over the years. Quite honestly, if I taught the same postures with the same instructions over and over again in all my classes, it would get boring, if not for my students, at the very least for myself. Without any variation in my chosen posture sequences, I also would not have been able to sustain my own regular practice for the last six years. The point being is that it is so very important to keep your yoga practice fresh, adding novelty and movement to pique your interest. It might be analogous to eating the same entree each time you go to your favorite restaurant that hasn't changed its menu for years.

Without trying something new, the possibility of instilling new vigor into your life experiences is nonexistent. I might try a new variation of an *asana*. Two possibilities exist: I experience a new wonderful stretch that I had never appreciated before or I find the new variation just doesn't feel good. Regardless of either outcome, through experimentation my mind was actively considering new perspectives. My thoughts were dedicated solely to this novel experience, rather than to what I needed to pick up at the supermarket or, even worse, to negative self-judgments and rumination.

The following is intended to illustrate how to introduce novelty into a posture sequence. Through the art of learned relaxation, however, you can tap into your own creativity to add new and innovative ways of positioning the body to any of these posture sequences or any *asana* you choose. Be inquisitive in your own unique version of yoga in which you not only change the position of the physical body, but also your way of thinking. In yoga, you are in control of your own experience, both physically and spiritually.

I. Begin in **tadasana,** the mountain pose. As always, activate the body by grounding into the mat. Let a wave of elongation spread up the spine to the crown of head. Bring the arms slightly away from your sides, palms facing forward. With your next deep inhalation, rotate just the right palm to face behind you. As you exhale, simultaneously rotate the right palm forward and the left palm to face behind you. Continue this alternation of the position of the palms connected to your breath. Deepen and slow the breath to slow down the rotation of the hands. When you are ready, bring both palms to face forward, close the eyes, take a deep breath and notice if your thoughts were in the moment and dedicated solely to your movements.

2. Relax the body and bring the hands to the hips. Find a *drishti*, deepen your breath, and bring all your weight onto one foot. Come into **utthita hasta padangusthasana variation**, the standing *crane pose,* arms at shoulder height and either balancing on toes or the big toe of the other foot or lifting the knee up towards the level of the hips. You will likely lift the arms to shoulder height in a habitual fashion. Now, simply bend the index finger of one hand on a deep inhalation. With a long exhalation, simultaneously extend the bent finger and bend the index finger on the opposite hand. Continue to connect the alternating flexion and extension of the fingers to the breath. Introduction of movement into an ordinarily static balance posture creates a novel point of focus that diverts attention away from concerns of physical balance. Connecting a deep breath to the movement triggers the relaxation response, which softens muscles and facilitates

physical balance. If you do wobble or fall out of this pose, simply return back to your version of the standing crane pose. Multiple attempts do not cost anything. As in life, a desired goal isn't necessarily realized on the first attempt. Try the posture with the weight supported by the other leg. You can experiment with different movements to see if they change your experience. For example, you could alternate flexing and extending each wrist with each inhalation and exhalation.

3. Once both feet have returned to the ground, rotate 90 degrees to face the long edge of the mat and take a large step apart with the feet. Sweep the arms up into your star, ***utthita tadasana.*** With inhalation, pull widespread fingers away from the body and ground feet into the mat to energize the arms and legs. With exhalation, release the stretch in the arms and the contraction of the leg muscles, experiencing a release of energy. Slow down your breathing as you continue to pulsate between activation and release with each inhalation and exhalation. Once again, conscious thought and awareness are required in converting this ordinarily static posture into a dynamic one.

4. When you are ready, inhale into the energy of your star, but now with exhalation, bend elbows and knees to sink into ***utkata konasana,*** the goddess

pose. Once again, slow down your breathing as you continue to rise into the star with inhalation and sink into the goddess with exhalation. Allow the breath to direct the movement. Enjoy the slow flow as you harness the energy of your star to fuel the power of your goddess.

5. Return to the star and lower both arms to shoulder height. Rotate one foot and the head 90 degrees. Bend the front knee into *virabhadrasana II*, warrior II. Activate the legs and arms. Create minimal, almost imperceptible, movement of the hips front and back. Inhale the hips forward, exhale them back to convert a familiar static posture into an interesting, dynamic one. Bring the hips to stillness. With a single point of focus on your front hand, bend the index finger. Once again, it is close to impossible for all of your attention not to be directed to that single deliberate movement.

6. Now let the subtle movements in warrior II become more expansive as you inhale into *viparita virabhadrasana,* the reverse warrior, and exhale into *utthita parsvakonasana,* the extended angle, passing through the warrior on your excursion between the two poses. Let the windmilling of the arms between the two *asanas* be fluid and graceful. Perhaps flex and extend the wrists and move fingers as the arms float back and forth, as if you are a tree with its

branches swaying in a soft breeze. See if the movement can be continuous, not stopping at either end of the flow.

7. Return to warrior II. Rotate the front foot ninety degrees and bring your hands to your hips. With feet parallel or slightly pigeon-toed, hinge over at the hips with a flat back into **prasarita padottanasana**, the wide angle standing forward fold. Begin to create slight rocking movements of the hips. Inhale the hips to one side and exhale to the other. Experiment with larger excursions of the hips from side to side, shifting weight from one foot to the other.

8. Return to center and gradually bring your torso back upright. Exiting from an inversion, a posture where the head is below the heart, must be done slowly to prevent orthostatic hypotension i.e. keeping the blood in the brain.

9. You can repeat steps five through seven with warrior II on the other side. Experiment with other body movements to make the flow your own personal experience.

10. Return to *tadasana*. Take a large sun breath with a deep inhalation. With exhalation, swan dive down into a standing forward fold. With your next inhalation, plant your hands and step back into **adho mukha svanasana**, downward facing dog. Once

again, find movement in the posture, possibly peddling feet or swaying hips. Regardless of whether your movements are subtle or gross, always make sure that they are connected to the breath. Slower movements and deeper breathing better induce feelings of relaxation.

11. Finally, drop your knees and push back into **balasana**, the child's pose. As always, make sure to support the forehead to remove any stress from the neck and shoulders. Relax the body and find your way into stillness. Digest your experience with self-inquiry.

HONORING THE SPINE

- *Tadasana ~ The Mountain*
- *Indudalasana ~ Standing Half Crescent Moon Pose*
- *Uttanasana ~ Standing Forward Fold*
- *Bitilasana ~ The Cow Pose*
- *Marjaryasana ~ The Cat Pose*
- *Salamba Bhujangasana ~ The Sphinx Pose*
- *Bhujangasana ~ The Cobra Pose*
- *Urdhva Mukha Svanasana ~ Upward Facing Dog*
- *Balasana ~ Child's Pose*
- *Matsyendrasana ~ Seated Spinal Twist*

- *Setu Bandhasana ~ Bridge Pose*
- *Supta Matsyendrasana ~ Supine Spinal Twist*

The spine is important from both physical and spiritual perspectives. Many of the *chakras,* the *sushumna nadi,* and the *ida* and *pingala nadis* are all intimately associated with the spine. This energy system was one of the earliest attempts to describe human anatomy and physiology, and as such, represents a true marvel. In many ways, the ideas put forth by the ancient yogis are not dissimilar to the actual anatomy of the nervous system as we know it today.

I refer you back to the chapter on The Love of Wisdom and The Love of Self for a more detailed description of the *chakras.* As you progress through this posture sequence and explore each *chakra,* breathe deeply into any personal meanings and positive affirmations that arise from fueling the energy of each one. As was discussed, each *chakra* governs the energy for qualities of the human condition that we strive to possess:

- *Root chakra ~ safety and security*
- *Sacral chakra ~ creativity*
- *Solar plexus chakra ~ power, wisdom and strength*
- *Heart chakra ~ love, compassion and gratitude*
- *Throat chakra ~ expression*
- *Third eye chakra ~ insight and connection*
- *Crown of head chakra ~ spirituality*

The intention of this book is to present ways to cope with depression and anxiety through the practice of yoga. An integral part of that practice is embracing self-kindness by substituting positive affirmations for automatic negative thoughts. The brain listens to everything you tell it. Imagine that you are having a discussion with an interested good friend about the *chakras.* Can you ask your friend about a time or times in life when he, she or they experienced the energy of the *chakras:* feeling safe and secure, creative, powerful, wise and strong, and loving, compassionate and grateful? The answer requires tapping into the energies of the throat *chakra* and the third eye for one to clearly express insight into these emotions and human qualities. The final result is the flow of energy into the crown of head with an elevation of the spirit though the introduction of positive affirmations. Allow that interested good friend to be yourself.

The following posture sequence employs all six movements of the spine: flexion, extension, right and left lateral flexion and right and left twisting. Yoga affords the wonderful opportunity to connect the physical and spiritual by linking your own images of the activation of the *chakras* with your movements, thereby focusing the mind on ideas that exist in the present. Once again, the art of learned relaxation is based in your imagination and creativity.

1. Begin in ***tadasana,*** the mountain pose, facing the front of the mat. The Sanskrit word "chakra" means

"wheel". As you ground into the mat, imagine a surge of energy spreading up the *sushumna nadi,* the main energy channel, causing each wheel to spin and emit the energy specific to each *chakra.* Each *chakra* is also assigned a color of the rainbow, ranging from red for the root to violet for the crown of head. You might also breathe deeply into the color of each *chakra* to intensify the color of its light.

2. Place your hand on your hip. Press the hip away to one side to shift your weight onto the opposite-sided foot, while you sweep your arm overhead and over, stretching fingertips to the other side to create the crescent shape of **indudalasana**, the standing crescent moon pose. Breathe into the stretch along the side body. This *asana* employs two of the movements of the spine: lateral flexion to the right and left. A wonderful way to experience *indudalasana* is to alternately arch from one side to the other, connecting the breath to a graceful, fluid undulating movement of the arms and hands, as if they are branches of a willow tree blowing in the breeze. Enjoy the changing shapes and the cooling energy of your crescent moon.

3. Inhale the arms overhead. Pause to enjoy a full body stretch, feeling your spine lengthening. Slowly exhale to swan dive into **uttanasana**, the standing forward fold. This posture requires flexion

or a bending forward of the spine. Remain in *uttanasana* for as long as you wish, sinking into this passive posture.

4. When you feel ready, plant the hands, step back into downward facing dog, drop the knees and come into a table position. **Bitilasana**, the cow, and **marjaryasana**, the cat, are almost always done concurrently as complementary poses. One transitions from back extension in the cow pose to back flexion in the cat pose. Sinking into a meditative state is potentiated by closing the eyes and letting the breath direct the movement. By removing visual stimuli, one can better focus on what is happening in the body, including an awareness of the connection of breath to movement. In that regard, create and link two waves. One is the breath that begins at the bottom of the belly and progresses to the upper chest with full inhalation and then returns in the opposite direction with a long exhalation. The other wave is the movement of the body. Enter into the cow pose, allowing the inhalation to first lift the tailbone. The chest and head lift as the breath progresses into the upper chest. The wave of exhalation drops the head, rounds the back and drops the tailbone. Focus on the two, intimately connected waves

progressing from tailbone to head and returning from head to tailbone.

5. The next three postures are all back bends involving back extension of varying degrees of intensity. From the table position, slide your legs back as you come to lie on your belly, head supported by chin or forehead. Bring the elbows directly under the shoulders, forearms and palms face down on the mat. Ground the tops of feet, thighs, pelvis, forearms and hands into the mat as you press up with an arched back into **salamba bhujangasana**, the sphinx pose. Inhale deeply into the back bend, then slowly lower the chest and head back toward the mat with exhalation, releasing the activation of the body and breathing out the energy of the pose.

6. Bring the hands at or just below the shoulders and hug the ribs with the forearms. Ground the tops of feet, thighs, and pelvis into the mat as you press up and arch the back into **bhujangasana**, the cobra pose. Make sure to continue to hug the ribs with your arms and breathe deeply as you lift chest and gaze up. Inhale deeply into the back bend, exhale to lower the chest and head to the mat, once again releasing the energy of the pose.

7. With the next inhalation, press into the hands firmly to lift the pelvis off of the mat, coming into

our last back bend, ***urdhva mukha svanasana,***
upward facing dog. Allow the hips to become heavy
and sag with gravity like a hammock to intensify
back extension. Inhale deeply into the back bend.
Exhale the body back down to the mat, release and
relax.

8. After three back extension poses, it is time for a
counterpose to balance extension with flexion. This
is achieved by pushing back into **balasana**, the
child's pose. Child's pose balances activity with
stillness. We can be aware of the physical body by
breathing deeply into the rounding of the back. We
can also breathe into thoughts, ideas and emotions.
The breath occurs in the present, diverting
attention away from thoughts that don't. In the
practice of yoga, we are always striving for
mindfulness of the moment to elicit relaxation and
a sense of wellbeing. The child's pose affords you
time to think. You might take this time to return to
the imagery of the wheels of energy of the *chakras*
glowing brightly with the colors of the rainbow.
Allow each long exhalation to slow down the
spinning of the wheels and enjoy the peacefulness
of calming stillness.

9. Take your time to come to sit on your mat. For
Matsyendrasana, the seated spinal twist, the inside
of one foot, say the right, is brought next to the

inside of the left thigh. Grab the right knee with the left hand or left elbow and windmill the right arm over and behind you as you twist. Bring your gaze over the right shoulder. Breathe deeply. You will notice that it is more difficult to inhale in a twisted position. With each inhalation, actively pull the right thigh into the belly to lengthen the spine. With each exhalation, see if there is a little more that the spine can twist each time. Finally, activate the extended left leg by pushing its heel away. When you are ready, untwist the torso and repeat the posture on the other side. Notice if one side feels different than the other. Much asymmetry exists in the apparent symmetry of our bodies.

10. Lower your back onto the mat. With knees bent, soles of the feet on the mat, arms at your sides and palms face down, walk your heels close to your sitz bones. Deeply inhale the hips upwards to come into **setu bandhasana**, the bridge pose. I find the bridge pose becomes a much more meditative experience by introducing motion into the posture. With each inhalation lift the hips upwards and the arms overhead. As you exhale, drop the hips and return the arms back to your sides. Let this upward and downward motion become your own graceful flow by extending and flexing the wrists as the arms float up and down.

Slow the breath to slow down the motion. Inhale to lift the hips and arms, grounding firmly into the mat with both feet as you stretch your fingertips away from the body. Release all tension of the body as you exhale and enjoy a feeling of weightlessness as the hips and arms float back down to the ground.

11. The bridge creates back extension. Grab knees to the chest to flex or round the back as a counterpose. With knees remaining bent toward the chest, release the arms to the ground at shoulder height and let the knees drop to one side to come into *supta Matsyendrasana*, the supine spinal twist. Surrender into this posture. Let the body become heavy and sink into the mat with each exhalation. We wish to remove all physical tension while assuming this pose. If the knees do not touch the ground, readjust the legs into a more comfortable position. Come into stillness and bring your awareness to a deep breath. Repeat on the opposite side.

12. It is easy to transition from the supine spinal twist into *shavasana* by bringing knees to center and extending the legs. *Shavasana* is your time to just be. For a few moments, give yourself permission to release whatever might be pressing down on your spirit and simply relax. Imagine the spinning

chakras gradually slowing to a stop. At this moment there is nothing to do and nowhere to be.

LESS IS MORE

- *Bharmasana ~ Table Pose*
- *Bitilasana ~ The Cow Pose*
- *Marjaryasana ~ The Cat Pose*
- *Balasana ~ Child's Pose*
- *Urdhva Mukha Svanasana ~ Upward Facing Dog*
- *Bharmasana ~ Table Pose*
- *Windshield-Wipering the Legs*
- *Setu Bandhasana ~ The Bridge Pose*
- *Supta Matsyendrasana ~ Supine Spinal Twist*
- *Shavasana*

The intention of this posture sequence is to do less with the physical body to create more time to sink into contemplative thought. As in life, sometimes having a realistic expectation to do less can paradoxically increase your ability to do more. A pressure to accomplish everything at once can leave one flustered with less focus and concentration. Alternatively, taking one step at a time can increase productivity and chances for success.

Sometimes, a slower paced practice with a greater

emphasis on the breath can be a more effective reducer of stress than a more vigorous, fast moving posture sequence. Similar to all of the other posture sequences, this one promotes inwardness through a connection of breath to movement, but its slower pace fosters a greater connection to self. Quite simply, a slower pace gives you more time to think.

As you practice this posture sequence, take the time in each *asana* to allow the breath to wash over your body with waves of relaxation. Let each inhalation fill your body with positive energy and, with each exhalation, allow your body to surrender and sink into the mat. Our goal is for slow movements and transitions between poses. Less movement translates to more time for self-discovery.

1. Start in **bharmasana**, the table pose. Become mindful of the contact points of the body on the mat. Spread your fingers wide such that the palm also contacts the mat. Imagine your hands are like suction cups on the mat. Now, come into *dirga pranayama* by establishing a long, deep breath that begins at the bottom of the belly and spreads like a wave to the top of the chest. Stay here breathing as long as you wish.

2. When you are ready to create movement, slowly come into **bitilasana**, the cow pose, and **marjaryasana**, the cat pose. Imagine a gentle wave approaching the shore. That wave begins with the

lifting of the tailbone, followed by the arching of
the back and, finally, by the lifting of the chest and
head. The wave ebbs out to sea by first dropping the
head, rounding the back and, finally, tucking the
tailbone. Now, connect the wave of your breath to
the wave of your movement. As you deepen and
slow the breath, slow down the movement.
Remember, there is no rush. Closing the eyes will
heighten awareness of the connection of the two
waves. Perhaps, sustain each posture by inserting a
pause at full inhalation and another at complete
exhalation or see if you can seamlessly transition
from the cow to cat and cat to cow without stopping
in either pose. If you find that this interplay
between breath and movement is relaxing, you may
wish to continue, gracefully transitioning from cow
and cat, for a longer duration.

3. When you are ready, push back into **balasana**,
   child's pose. Rest here for as long as you wish,
   breathing deeply to round the back. Child's pose is
   one of stillness and reflection. As such, we wish to
   reduce physical tension to lose awareness of the
   physical body. As it bears repeating, it is important
   to support the forehead. The head weighs ten to
   fifteen pounds. Letting it float in space puts stress
   on the neck and shoulders. Child's pose affords a
   wonderful opportunity to connect with thoughts

and feelings. The content of thoughts may seem difficult to control at times. It is fine if that happens. At the very least, while in child's pose, you can let a deep breath trigger the parasympathetic response, as relaxation takes hold in subconscious thought.

4. When you are ready to emerge from the stillness of child's pose, as if you are moving in slow motion, begin to slide forward into **urdhva mukha svanasana**, upward facing dog. Push into both palms and let the hips sag downward to accentuate the arch in the back. Find *dirga pranayama*. On your next long exhalation, push back into child's pose. As you inhale, push slowly forward into upward facing dog. Continue this back and forth flow. The degree of arching and rounding of the back between this pose and counterpose will be a magnitude greater than the cow and cat. Connect the wave of slow, deep breathing to the wave of movement. Let the breath, not conscious thought, direct your movements. The slower the breath, the slower the movement. Once again, continue this flow for as long or short as you wish.

5. Return to **bharmasana**, the table pose. Swing your legs foward to come to sit on your mat. With hands behind your back and knees bent, place your feet to the outer edges of your mat. **Windshield-wiper your knees** from one side to the other. Notice how

you may be habitually moving your legs rather quickly back and forth. Bring awareness once again to the breath. Inhale the knees to one side and exhale them to the other. The slower and deeper the breath, the slower the movement of the legs becomes. Close your eyes and let breath and movement become one.

6. When you feel ready, lower the back onto your mat. With knees bent, push your hips up into *setu bandhasana*, the bridge pose. You can sustain this posture or create an up-and-down movement of the hips connected to a slow and deep breath. If you have a block, you can place it at its lowest setting to support the sacrum to assume a supported bridge, a restorative pose that involves a gentle, passive stretch of the muscles of the back.

7. After exiting *setu bandhasana,* use your feet and hands to shift your hips to one edge of your mat. Bring arms into a "T-shape" at shoulder height on the ground. Draw knees to the chest and let them fall to the side to enter into *supta Matsyendrasana*, the supine spinal twist. If the knees do not comfortably reach the ground, readjust the legs into any configuration necessary to release tension. Surrender into this pose. Let each exhalation pull the body into the mat. When you feel ready, repeat on the other side.

8. Bring the knees to center, extend out the legs and bring the arms to your sides. The supreme relaxation of *shavasana* awaits you.

CREATING BALANCE

- *Dirga Pranayama in Stillness with Hands in Anjali Mudra at Heart Center*
- *Vrikshasana ~ The Tree Pose*
- *Dirga Pranayama in Stillness with Hands in Anjali Mudra at Heart Center*
- *Utthita Hasta Padangusthasana Variation ~ Standing Crane Pose*
- *Dirga Pranayama in Stillness with Hands in Anjali Mudra at Heart Center*
- *Garudasana ~ The Eagle Pose*
- *Dirga Pranayama in Stillness with Hands in Anjali Mudra at Heart Center*
- *Natarajasana ~ The Lord of the Dance or Dancer's Pose*
- *Dirga Pranayama in Stillness with Hands in Anjali Mudra at Heart Center*
- *Eka pada utkatasana ~ Standing Figure Four Pose*
- *Dirga Pranayama in Stillness with Hands in Anjali Mudra at Heart Center*
- *Virabhadrasana III ~ Warrior III*

- *Dirga Pranayama in Stillness with Hands in Anjali Mudra at Heart Center*

This posture sequence consists of a series of balance postures and alternating periods of rest and reflection. A primary goal of yoga is to create a balance. We strive to balance mind and body. We strive to balance *prana,* the life-force, throughout all of the *nadis,* or energy channels, of the body by controlling the breath. We strive to create a balance of the feminine, cooling, and insightful energy of the *ida nadi* and the masculine, active and impulsive energy of the *pingala nadi.* We strive to balance the sympathetic and parasympathetic nervous systems. Rather than being stuck in chronic anxiety-related sympathetic overload, we wish the sympathetic response to be situationally appropriate. Increasing parasympathetic tone induces states of relaxation.

More so than any of the other *asanas,* balance postures require single-pointed focus to achieve physical stability. The single visualized object of observation is called a *drishti. Drishti* is a Sanskrit word meaning "a focused gaze". It is a chosen point on the floor, wall, in nature or on the horizon on which to concentrate. Although we try to practice non-attachment to outcomes in yoga, if one must define success in a balance posture, it is not the ability to stand on one leg. Rather, it is the ability to have single-pointed concentration in order to clear the mind of all other thoughts. Arguably, one with a clear mind with both feet on the ground has a greater mastery of a balance posture than one who is wobbling on one leg, their mind clouded by the struggle to physically balance. The *drishti* is not something to stare at, but rather something to observe. Deliberate inquiry into the qualities and characteristics of your *drishti* enhances clarity of mind. Even more so, breathing deeply into your *drishti* can transport you into the present, imaging your point of observation being drawn closer to you with each deep inhalation.

This posture sequence is about teaching the brain to be in the moment. Inherent to depression and anxiety is a tendency for rumination, which is lessened by creating clarity of mind that comes from living in the present.

As you progress through this posture sequence, bear in mind that using a wall or prop or resting toes on the mat are wonderful options to aid in establishing physical stability. Remember that options are not challenges. If lifting the foot off of the mat without the use of a wall or prop creates imbalance, then the mind will be flooded with thoughts of instability, layered with potential negative self-judgments about an inability to physically balance on one leg. It is all about perspective. What is the goal for which we strive in a balance posture? Is it achieving physical balance or mental clarity? Arguably, the latter is much more difficult to achieve. Learning to be in the moment and quieting the mind of thoughts that don't serve is the work to be done in any attempt to balance, either on one leg or throughout life.

The *asanas* presented here in this sequence become

progressively more physically challenging. Once again, props or a wall can help you better handle the more advanced postures. Feel free to substitute and repeat postures that seem more reasonable for your present physical abilities. As a yoga instructor, I am merely a guide. I make suggestions that I believe can enhance your practice, but never feel compelled to do anything I suggest. Yoga is a personal experience. More important than experiencing my version of yoga is to create your own version that best honors your body and mind.

Periods of stillness that separate the postures in this sequence are an opportunity for self-inquiry. You have time to ask yourself if you achieved heightened awareness of your *drishti* or, rather, what other thoughts occupied your mind that distracted you from physically balancing. Were those thoughts negative judgments about your inability to balance? Alternatively, with hands at heart center, the energy center for love, compassion and gratitude, you might create an image in the mind of someone or something for which you are grateful. Consider two individuals. One laments a failure to achieve physical balance. The other is filled with positive energy by recognizing their blessings. Yoga affords the time to decide the individual you wish to be.

1. Start in a passive standing position. Allow all your muscles to release and imagine the body to be weightless in space. Find a *drishti*, a point of focus on the floor, wall, or something that can be seen

from your window or out on the horizon. Come into
dirga pranayama, the complete yogic breath.
Imagine the *drishti* being drawn closer and closer
with each deep inhalation. Bring your hands to
your hips. Take a moment to rock from side to side
to notice weight shifting from one foot to the other.
Continue deep breathing as you shift all of your
weight onto one foot.

2. Ground your foot into the mat, imagine the
engaged leg to be the strong trunk of your tree, the
foot your roots. Inhale the heel of your other foot
up from the mat and exhale the heel onto the inside
of the opposite ankle, balancing on toes or just the
big toe. Inhale the arms up overhead with
outstretched fingers to create the branches of your
tree to arrive in *vrikshasana*, the tree pose.
Alternatively, hands can be brought together in
anjali mudra at heart center. Option to slide the sole
of the foot onto the inside of the calf or thigh. To
prevent knee injury, if falling out of the pose, never
rest the foot on the inside of the knee.

3. Deeply inhale, and then with a slow exhalation
gently release the pose. Close the eyes and find your
way into stillness with hands in *anjali mudra.* Re-
establish *dirga pranayama.*

4. Repeat step one. Then ground your foot into the
mat, imagine your leg to be that of a wading bird

standing motionless in a glade. Inhale the heel of the other foot up from the mat and rest the toes or the big toe on the mat. Raise the arms to shoulder height to create the outstretched wings of your bird as you enter into a variation of **utthita hasta padangusthasana,** standing crane pose. Option to lift the knee up toward the level of the hip. Option to flex the ankle, pushing the heel toward the ground and the toes upwards.

5. Release the pose, close the eyes and find your way into stillness with hands in *anjali mudra.* Re-establish *dirga pranayama.*

6. Repeat step one. For the full expression of **garudasana,** the eagle pose, legs and arms wrap into eagle legs and arms. Once again, many options exist to tailor this *asana* to best promote focus and concentration. Some options include the back of hands touch rather than the palms being brought together while in eagle arms, forearms crossed and palms resting on shoulders, or resting the non-weight bearing toes or big toe on the mat.

7. Release the pose, close the eyes and find your way into stillness with hands in *anjali mudra.* Re-establish *dirga pranayama.*

8. Repeat step one. **Natarajasana,** the Lord of the Dance or dancer's pose, requires grabbing the foot or ankle behind the buttocks, which is a challenge

of flexibility. One might first come into the standing crane and then draw the foot back into the hand. We strive to tap into our grace as we become the dancer, creating beautiful arcs in the back and the arm lifted up toward the sky.

9. Release the pose, close the eyes and find your way into stillness with hands in *anjali mudra*. Re-establish *dirga pranayama*.

10. Repeat step one. **Eka pada utkatasana**, standing figure four pose, requires crossing the ankle on to the thigh of the standing leg while sitting down on an imaginary chair. Hands can be held in *anjali mudra* at heart center.

11. Release the pose, close the eyes and find your way into stillness with hands in *anjali mudra*. Re-establish *dirga pranayama*.

12. Repeat step one. From warrior I, shift weight onto the front foot. Hinge forward at the hips creases while extending arms forward to come into **virabhadrasana III**, warrior III. This represents a physically challenging pose. Supporting a hand on a block can facilitate balance.

13. Release the pose, close the eyes and find your way into stillness with hands in *anjali mudra*. Re-establish *dirga pranayama*.

14. Repeat this entire posture sequence or whatever portion you chose to do with weight supported on

the other leg. Notice if your experience changes
from one side of the body to the other.

Looking back at this posture sequence, which are the most important steps? The answer, of course, are all of the odd numbered steps. A balance posture should never be considered a physical challenge, but rather a mental challenge to achieve a single point of focus. As bears repeating: arguably, a person who achieves that focus with both feet on the ground is more successful than the person who wobbles while attempting to stand on one leg, their mind clouded with the experience of physical instability. The latter person's experience is worsened if he, she or they, while standing in stillness, laments their inability to achieve physical balance. The emphasis should always be on whatever promotes self-kindness, which in this posture sequence is facilitated by experiencing hands in *anjali mudra* at heart center, the energy center for love, compassion and gratitude.

As you repeat this sequence on the opposite side, remove any pressure to perform. De-emphasize the physical postures and focus on quieting the mind and finding relaxation in your times of stillness. This book is all about making choices. Choose self-compassion and accept yourself as you are.

FEET FIRST

- *Tadasana ~ The Mountain*
- *Indudalasana ~ Standing Half Crescent Moon Pose*
- *Utkatasana ~ The Chair Pose*
- *Virabhadrasana II ~ Warrior II*
- *Utthita tadasana ~ The Star*
- *Utkata Konasana ~ The Goddess Pose*
- *Virabhadrasana I ~ Warrior I*
- *Buddha virabhadrasana ~ The Humble Warrior*
- *Balasana ~ Child's Pose*

The name of this posture sequence might sound intriguing or a bit unusual, but the position of and weight distribution on the feet dictates the position of the remainder of the body for all of our standing *asanas*. As you progress through this posture sequence, a heightened awareness of the feet can serve as the single-pointed focus for which we continually strive as we practice the learned art of relaxation. Four conditions exist with regard to the feet:

1. *Position of the feet and their relationship on the mat ~* for example, aligned or spaced out wide apart.
2. *The weight distribution ~* whether the body weight is supported by the entire foot or weight is shifted to one part of the foot, such as the ball or heel, or

weight is shifted on onto one foot while the other bears no body weight.

3. *Grounding* ~ simply put, applying a downward force on the feet through engagement of the muscles of the legs, establishing the important connection of self to the earth below.

4. *Softening of the feet* ~ essentially relaxing the leg muscles to minimize the weight bearing of both feet

For this posture sequence, bringing one's awareness to the conditions of the feet clears the mind of other thoughts that don't serve in the moment; the goal of meditation.

We will consider the four conditions above as they relate to *tadasana*, the mountain. First, the position of the feet are such that they are parallel under the hips, approximately 6-8 inches apart. Second, in *tadasana*, the body weight is evenly distributed on all parts of the foot from toes to heel. Take a moment to slightly rock forward and back, sensing the change in weight distribution, then find a point of rest where all parts of the bottom of the foot are evenly bearing weight. Next we begin to ground the feet into the mat and notice the contraction of the leg muscles. As we apply the downward force, energy develops in the opposite direction causing an elongation of the spine; our mountain standing strong and tall. Finally, soften the feet by relaxing the body, especially the leg muscles, coming into stillness and allowing yourself to reflect on the experience of *tadasana*.

1. Start in *tadasana*, as described above. Once you have engaged the legs, with arms at your sides, begin to spread fingers wide, pulling them towards the earth. I like to cup my hands and angle them slightly skyward, as if I am receiving a small bit of the energy of the universe.

2. With your next deep inhalation, pull the fingers outward and upwards. As the palms meet, interlace the fingers.For *indudulasna*, the feet remain parallel, 6-8 inches apart. Now, shift the hips to one side, let us say the right, as all of the body weight comes onto the right foot. Now take the vertical line of energy from *tadasana* and bend it to the left, arching over to the left and pulling fingers to the left to counteract the rightward force in the hips. Return to center, noticing all the weight returning to both feet, then repeat the standing half crescent moon pose on the other side with a heightened awareness of the shift of weight to the left foot.

3. Return back to center, release the interlace of the fingers and bring both arms down to shoulder height in front of you, palms face down. Begin pulling your fingers foward such that the body weight shifts forward onto the balls and toes of the feet, as if a nice friend is trying to pull you forward off of your mat. Now, bend your knees and pull your hips down and back and notice the weight rolling

from the balls and toes back onto the heels, as you enter into **utkatasana**, the chair pose. In the chair pose, all of the body weight is supported by the heels, enabling you to wiggle the toes to demonstrate that this is the case. Balancing the body weight on the heels can leave you in a precarious position. Stability comes from counteracting the backward pull of the hips with the frontward force of your outstretched arms.

4. Drop your arms behind you to come into a deeper crouch and the downhill skier's position. With your next deep breath in, sweep the arms overhead as you come to stand erect. Let the hands come together in *anjali mudra.* As you exhale, let the palms come down to heart center. Let the body become soft and feel the feet become lighter as the body weight minimally presses downward. Come into stillness and digest the experience.

5. Come to the front of your mat. Swing one leg, say the left leg, behind the other to enter into **virabhadrasana II**, warrior II. The difference between *virabhadrasana* I and II lies in the position of the feet. The feet position dictates what the rest of the body is doing. In *virabhadrasana II*, the feet line up as if you are standing on a balance beam. A line drawn from the front heel should intersect the arch of the perpendicular back foot. This feet

position allows for the the hips and chest to rotate to the side as is found in the full expression of the pose. For *virabhadrasana I*, the feet are spaced apart as if you are standing on railroad tracks. This allows for the hips and shoulders to face forward. Before moving onto the star pose, experience the strength of your warrior II, as you ground your feet into the mat to activate the leg muscles to create a strong stable base. Stretch the arms in opposite directions to form a straight line of energy from fingertips to fingertips. Now, rotate the front right foot ninety degrees and the back left foot ninety degrees to arrive in your warrior II on the other side. Once again, energize your warrior.

6. Straighten your front leg and rotate the front foot ninety degrees, such that both feet are parallel, toes pointing forward. Splay your feet to forty-five degree angles and sweep your arms upward to forty-five degree angles to come into **utthita tadasana**, the star pose. Ground your feet downward as you pull your fingers outward to create four lines of energy that radiate like a star from your solar plexus *chakra*, the energy center for power and wisdom. It is your wisdom that allows you to reflect on past experiences and to apply what you have learned to future possibilities. It is your power that

allows you to face any challenges that may lie in those possibilities.

7. Bend the knees and elbows to come into **utkata konasana**, the goddess pose. Bring awareness to your feet. As you press downward, allow the downward force to elongate the legs to flow back into the star. As you release the force on the feet, sink back down into your goddess. Enjoy this flow of activation and release for as long as you wish.

8. When you are ready, heel-toe your feet together and go to the back of your mat. Once again, bring awareness to the feet. Begin with legs out wide, imagining you are standing on two train tracks. Take a big step forward, let's say with the right foot, as if you are stepping through a doorway into a room, possibly imagining it to be your beautiful sanctuary that you create in your mind, and seeing it clearly with the third eye *chakra*, the energy center for insight. Although you have stepped forward, your feet should remain widely spaced, remaining on those two train tracks, enabling the hips and shoulders to face forward. You have stepped forward into **virabhadrasana I**, the warrior I. Ground your feet into the mat to engage the legs as you stretch the arms upward in the opposite direction to fuel both your physical and inner warrior.

9. Bring the palms together. Deeply inhale. As you slowly exhale, allow the hands to drift down to heart center. Hinge forward at the hip creases with a flat back into **buddha virabhadrasana**, the humble warrior. To counteract the upper body weight shifting forward, ground firmly with the back foot, such that weight remains evenly distributed on both feet. Perhaps, with a heightened awareness of the feet, rock slightly forward and back to appreciate the shifting weight. Settle on a place where the weight is evenly distributed. Think of the legs as the pedestal of a statue. Regardless of the position that the upper body assumes, the pedestal is immovable. Repeat the warrior I and humble warrior on the other side.

10. Finally, bring your hands to frame your front foot. Step back into high plank. Drop you knees and push back into a well deserved rest in **balasana**, the child's pose. Perhaps, breathe deeply into the contact points of your body on the mat, which can become your single-point of focus on which to meditate.

THE POSTURE SEQUENCE OF SELF-KINDNESS

- *Sukhasana ~ The Easy Pose*
- *Adho Mukha Svanasana ~ Downward Facing Dog*
- *Phalakasana ~ Plank*
- *Vasisthasana ~ Side Plank*
- *Chaturanga Dandasana ~ Low Pushup*
- *Urdhva Mukha Svanasana ~ Upward Facing Dog*
- *Balasana ~ Child's Pose*
- *Adho Mukha Svanasana ~ Downward Facing Dog*
- *Phalakasana ~ Plank*
- *Vasisthasana ~ Side Plank*
- *Chaturanga Dandasana ~ Low Pushup*
- *Urdhva Mukha Svanasana ~ Upward Facing Dog*
- *Balasana ~ Child's Pose*

On the face of it, this posture sequence might seem physically challenging and you might wonder how it could possibly be a practice of self-kindness. When considering this posture sequence, however, perhaps physically challenging *asanas* can serve as a metaphor for the daily challenges stemming from mental illness. Overcoming them is not necessarily easy. We can be kind to ourselves, however, by making modifications in our daily lives that make coping that much easier. It may be that we try to avoid uncomfortable anxiety-inducing situations and dysfunctional relationships that can make coping so much more onerous or establish boundaries from narcissistic and/or abusive people.

Being kind to yourself is treating yourself with compassion and self-respect to avoid doing harm to the spirit. Analogous to modifying your behaviors in difficult life situations, this posture sequence is practicing self-kindness by modifying any of the *asanas* to avoid any physical or mental discomfort, especially those that elicit negative self-judgments regarding perceived physical limitations.

Just like an empathetic friend that helps and supports you, be a friend to yourself. Support comes in many forms. In yoga, an important source of support are props. Yoga props include blocks, straps, blankets, bolsters and walls. If you are practicing at home and don't own yoga blocks or a bolster, a pillow or rolled up blanket are good alternatives. If you are considering a regular, at home yoga practice, however, I would suggest investing in yoga props, which you will find are readily available and relatively inexpensive online.

When I first began practicing yoga, I had the misconception that props were crutches to compensate for my limited abilities. When I went to yoga classes, it seemed like no one else was using props. Given my unhealthy attitude of self-competitiveness and a need to compare myself to others, I felt if I used props I was magnifying my physical limitations and ineptitude in the eyes of everyone else. My mind was clouded by self-deprecating thoughts. Eventually and fortunately, I learned that props are wonderful tools to create comfort and steadiness in a posture, which lead to a healthier mindset. Here were two people: my old self, overly concerned with appearances at the expense of my mental state and inability to relax, and my new self, dedicated to honoring my body and mind with kindness by reaching out for support. I let go of the mental real estate dedicated to beating myself up over my perceived limitations. Don't shy away from props if no one else is using them. If you witnessed a fellow classmate using a block or bolster, would you judge them? Be proud of yourself for honoring and being kind to your body. You might go even further and consider props your good friends; always there to give you support and strength to keep you balanced and well-grounded.

Just as you can use props for support in yoga, make sure to reach out for support in coping with your mental challenges. There is no reason to do it alone. Support can come from many sources including family, friends, mental health professionals, support groups, and hotlines.

As you progress through this posture sequence, honor your mind by accepting limitations. No one is perfect. No one is capable of everything. There is also no one that doesn't face challenges. Overcoming challenges is easier when you ask for support. As you perform this posture sequence, take time to consider if any of my suggested modifications enhances your experience by removing thoughts of discomfort that cloud the mind. Let those clouds disappear. If you can, as you progress through this posture sequence, try to deliberately affirm some positive attributes you possess. The brain listens to everything you tell it. Let it hear words of self-kindness and compassion.

This posture sequence is designed to emphasize modifications to the full expressions of these commonly practiced *asanas* in the interest of improved physical comfort, steadiness and strength. You might adopt the mantra, "I am being kind to myself" each time you modify a pose to best suit your body and mind, inhaling into "I am being " and exhaling, "kind to myself."

1. Begin in *sukhasana*, the easy pose, sitting with crossed legs. This is a misnomer for some, including myself, since this *asana* is not that easy. For me, because of tight inner thigh muscles and the innate structure of my pelvis, I sit in *sukhasasa* with my knees stuck way in the air way above my hips, causing my back to round. In fact, if you look around the room in a class, the knees of many of those in the easy pose are positioned above the hips. A consequent rounding of the back stresses muscles and crunches the abdominal contents, thereby preventing the full excursion of the diaphragm downward and limiting breathing capacity. By sitting on the edge of a bolster or cushion, the hips drop closer to or below the level of the hips with a consequent straightening of the spine and an increase of space in the abdomen for

greater downward excursion of the diaphragm, thereby optimizing breathing capacity. Here is your first opportunity in this posture sequence to practice self-kindness by using a prop in order to decrease discomfort and enhance your experience. You might experiment by experiencing *sukhasana* with and without a bolster to see which way feels best. Make sure to do a few rounds of deep diapraghmatic breathing in each option and notice which one allows you to take a deeper breath. In his *Yoga Sutras*, Pantanjali stressed sitting in a comfortable and steady position in which to perform *pranayama*. Always find your way into a posture that lessens the stress and tension on any part of your body. Release tension in the neck and shoulders by deeply inhaling your shoulders up to your ears and slowly exhaling to let the shoulder blades melt down the back. Come into several rounds of *dirga pranayama*. Bring your hands into *anjali mudra* at heart center and, with extreme self-kindness, honor yourself for being open to support. Honor yourself for taking the steps to overcome the challenges you face.

2. Take your time to transition into the table pose. Curl your toes and push the hips up and back to come into **adho mukha svanasana**, downward facing dog. In the ideal, full expression of this *asana*, the

soles of the feet are flat on the ground. For many of us, and possibly most of us, our heels cannot reach the floor and knees must bend. Once again, in the interest of practicing self-kindness, focus on what you can do and not what you can't. Let reality guide expectations. The only expression of a posture that is better than any other is one that best suits your body. Further, this pose for many, including myself, is not a comfortable one. I don't enjoy my head hanging down in space or sustained tension in my hamstrings. I often transition into a child's pose if I tire in a prolonged downward facing dog. Self-kindness is more easily practiced by accepting that not everything in yoga feels good. In life, similar realistic expectations can provide you with a healthier outlook.

3. Inhale deeply. As you exhale, draw your shoulders over your wrists and drop your hips to enter in *phalakasana*, high plank. Strength and stability come from actively pushing hands into the mat and pushing heels away from the body to induce a sense of full body tension. This is a physically demanding posture for many, so feel free to move on to step 4 at any time.

4. From the high plank, drop a knee, let's say the right, onto the mat directly under the right hip. Bring your right hand to center, directly under your nose.

As you rotate the right lower leg ninety degrees, perpendicular to the long edge of the mat, come onto the sole of the extended left foot and raise your left arm to the sky, coming into a supported side plank, or **vasisthasana**. Options include lifting the left leg or coming into a full side plank by extending out the right leg. Once again, use self-kindness to choose the option that is most steady and comfortable. One is not better than the other. Always remember that options are not challenges and yoga is not a competitive sport. Options are merely different ways to experience your yoga. Self-competitive judgments are wasted thoughts. Return to table position and repeat your version of side plank on the other side.

5. Return to table and step back into a high plank. Lower the body down to the mat with **charturanga dandasana**, the low pushup. As a modification, feel free to drop the knees onto the mat first to lessen the strain on the arms and shoulders as you lower your chest.

6. Transition into **urdhva mukha svanasana**, upward facing dog, by coming onto the tops of your feet and actively pushing through the hands to raise the hips. You could consider the option of lifting the knees off of the mat. These two options emphasize that yoga is a practice of personal decisions.

Connecting with yourself in order to analyze the implications of assuming a particular posture or any of its modifications leads to informed decisions about which variation of a pose best suits your physical body.

7. Push back into *balasana*, child's pose, and give yourself a present of a positive affirmation. Breathe into that thought and feel its energy spread throughout your body.

8. Slide forward into table position and repeat steps 2-7. As you do, honor yourself by exercising good judgment to choose the options that protect your body. Most importantly, in yoga and in life, be a good friend to yourself and practice self-kindness by modifying your experience to lessen the possibility of any harm to body and mind.

A posture sequence is like a road map that leads to your personal sanctuary. As with any destination, there are many different routes to get there. A posture sequence is not requisite to progress toward your goal. In the extreme, we needn't even consciously choose which *asana* to do. As such, consider the Kripalu yoga concept of *Meditation in Motion*. Through a regular practice of yoga, over time, the ability to access meditative states becomes so fine-tuned that rather than consciously entering into postures, the body moves spontaneously on a subconscious level. It is no longer the will of the mind that directs the movement of the body, but it is *prana,* the life force, that guides one through the postures. Removing conscious thoughts directed at specific movements of the body heightens the single-pointed concentration necessary for deep meditation and the converse; meditation is so deep that conscious thought is no longer needed for the movements of the body. When set to music, *Meditation in Motion* becomes a wonderful, flowing dance that engages mind and body with you as the choreographer.

As you might have noticed, each of the aforementioned posture sequences are not just a set of instructions to follow, but ways to actively participate in an exercise of mindfulness and self-exploration; one that requires creativity and engagement of the imagination. As a yoga instructor, I am not telling you that if you do a particular pose you should feel a certain way. Only you can know how something feels. It is for you to find out. In life, self-inquiry can better position you to choose that which best suits you, both on physical and emotional levels. You are free to explore possibilities to determine what lessens external stress and what doesn't. You are in control of choosing to pursue that which best promotes relaxation. And perhaps, the most important choice to make is that of self-kindness, in order to treat yourself with all the respect and worth that you deserve.

11

A TIME TO LET GO

Completely letting go is a state of being, devoid of any pressure to have to think or be anyone or anywhere. Up until this point, I have stressed the need to be focused on thoughts, ideas and physical sensations that are happening in the present moment to achieve states of relaxation. *Shavasana* is the one exception to that rule. It is typically assumed at the end of a yoga class, but can follow any of the posture sequences discussed in the prior chapter or serve as a single pose in which to fully release.

It is a slow, gradual descent into a place of peace that exists just below consciousness. As such, many feel that of all of the *asanas*, *shavasana* is the most challenging and difficult to master; more difficult than even the most physically demanding postures like headstands or standing splits. The true challenge of *shavasana* is achieving a complete loss of awareness of both body and mind. Arguably, the former is easier to achieve. A release of muscle tension follows deliberate softening of the physical body and implementing any changes in position that diminish any stress to muscles and joints. The latter is so much more difficult. Clearing the mind of all thoughts, either concrete or abstract, is a daunting challenge. In fact, I believe it is an unrealistic expectation that can lead to frustration. We are all fraught with mind chatter that varies in degree from day to day. At times, especially when it manifests as rumination on the despair and hopelessness inherent to mental disease, it can become all consuming. In *shavasana,* the best approach is to release all pressure to suppress mind chatter by recognizing that it is normal to have thoughts. A restful mind comes from acknowledging those thoughts as they arise, letting them disappear like a puff of smoke into the air and returning back to relaxation. In a sense, releasing thoughts in *shavasana* might be considered analogous to "thought stopping", a cognitive behavioral technique that can be useful to lessen anxiety.

I have also found that often while I am in *shavasana,* as well as during any meditative practice I might attempt, my mind wavers between stillness and active thinking. When I transition from the former to the latter and become conscious of thoughts, I find it to be a sought of awakening as I realize that I was in a meditative state for a period of time. I can relieve the pressure to achieve a quiet mind by embracing an active one. I am fine with and grateful for a modicum of quietude, even if it is just for a minority of the time.

Shavasana is traditionally done supine, legs extended, arms gently angled from the body, and palms face up. In yoga, palms facing toward the sky is considered a receptive posture. Although our desired goal is minimizing conscious thoughts, entering into *shavasana* receptive to new ideas and perspectives can maximize its benefits on a subconscious level. In the interest of eliminating any physical tension, however, the traditionally accepted pose may not necessarily be the most comfortable one. It might create less stress in the arms to lie with the palms face down or less stress on the lower back to have knees bent. Putting a bolster under the knees is a wonderful way to lessen any lower back strain. Some find more physical release in a fetal position or a supine spinal twist. Most important is to personalize your experience by assuming the most comfortable position that will allow you to lose awareness of the physical body.

Props can be helpful in finding a comfortable position for *shavasana*. A blanket over the body during *shavasana* can keep the body warm as it loses the heat generated by your physical practice. An eye pillow may eliminate any strain to keep the eyelids closed. Placing a rolled blanket under the neck can relieve tension in the cervical muscles and ligamentous and bony structures of the neck. Placing a bolster or block on the belly can create a sense of heaviness in the body that, for some, creates feelings of security.

Shavasana is an opportunity to allow yourself a few moments to rest the mind in a safe space. It is giving yourself permission to create distance from worries and stress through a realization that for a few moments nothing bad will happen if you just let go. Moreover, don't beat yourself up for failing to quiet your mind of chatter and unwanted thoughts on any particular day. Some days are different from others. If the mind remains active, at the very least, you are resting the body after a period of physical activity. For some, *shavasana* will induce sleep. Some say that falling asleep is the ultimate, highest level of relaxation. The hope is that you will arise from *shavasana* refreshed and energized with a healthier perspective to take on whatever lies ahead for the day.

Often in life we experience opposite extremes. Knowing the sensations and feelings evoked by one extreme gives one an appreciation for the other. The warmth of your home is much more evident when coming in from a cold, frigid day. The resting of the mind and body in *shavasana* is much more appreciated after a period of physical activity and engagement. Stretching and contracting muscles contrasts with physical release and relaxation. Strong emotions and profound ideas contrast with the stillness of the mind.

In my yoga classes, I end the period of *shavasana* by guiding my students back into awareness: of the breath by expanding belly and chest, of the physical body by initiating small movements that grow in size with each breath, and of their thoughts by awakening the mind. I then transition students from *shavasana* into a fetal position, a position of safety and rebirth. And as we emerge from the fetal pose, a wonderful metaphor can be considered: we are experiencing a rebirth into new exciting possibilities for a positive life filled with hope.

An important proviso is that for some who have suffered a prior trauma, closing their eyes in a room full of other people or lying supine with the sense that an instructor is watching can prove uncomfortable. Once again, like all of the other *asanas,* there are no hard and fast rules for *shavasana.* With eyes open, the body can still relax and the mind can be cleared by establishing a *drishti* on which to focus. It is important in a yoga class to always be in a safe space for both body and mind. Physical comfort can be also be achieved in a chair for those unable to come down on a mat. Yoga is a completely personal experience, uniquely performed by each one of us to best meet our individual needs.

Shavasana is an opportunity to rest the body and rest the mind. It is a few moments to give yourself permission to release the unwelcome weight of stressful or disturbing thoughts by saying that it is alright to simply just be. For those with mental disease, life can be a true battle. Sometimes, it is most beneficial to just stop fighting and call a ceasefire for a few moments to allow the mind and spirit to have a break from the stresses of life. In order to become free of the firm grasp of depression and anxiety, often it is necessary to let go of thoughts that press down upon the spirit and cloud the mind. *Shavasana* is that time to let go.

12

BREATHING INTO RELAXATION

U p until this point, we have considered the breath as an object of single-pointed focus and, when connected to one's unique ımovements, a vehicle to attain meditative states. Ultimately, awareness of the breath possesses the power to relax. We literally breathe into relaxation.

One can engage the senses to notice the sound of the breath, the alternating sensations of coolness and warmth in the nostrils with each inhalation and exhalation, or the expansion and contraction of the chest and abdomen with each breath. Connecting movements to the cycling of the breath induces feelings of inwardness.

I have previously described the physical action of diaphragmatic breathing as a trigger of the parasympathetic response. Out of danger, back in the safety of the cave, our caveman's breathing transitions from shallow, chest breaths initiated by the sympathetic system during the saber-toothed tiger attack to deep belly breaths that notify the brain and autonomic system that it is now time to rest and digest. Learning to consistently use the diaphragm to breathe also triggers the relaxation response over the long term. I am sure at one time or another someone observed you were stressed and told you to take a deep breath and relax. Further, you will observe many professional basketball players take a deep breath to relax the body and increase their focus right before attempting a free throw at the foul line. Deep breathing has a dual purpose: to promote feelings of inwardness and introversion through control and awareness and to induce the physiological-mediated relaxation response.

We can increase the relaxing and meditative power of the breath by dedicating our complete attention to the deliberate practice of specific breathing techniques. In yoga, these specific methods for eliciting breath-oriented states of relaxation are known as *pranayama;* a system that formalizes different ways of breathing that become the focus of mediation.

Pranayama necessitates not only an awareness, but also a control of the breath. In that regard, *"yama"* in the Sanskrit compound word, *pranayama,* translates to restraint or control. Of course, *prana* is considered the life force that surrounds us all and permeates the universe of which we are all a part. The aim of the yogic breathing techniques, therefore, is a control of the intake and balance of *prana*. In the context of this book's themes, however, *pranayama* serves as another tool to use in the art of learned relaxation.

Pranayama can be integrated into an *asana* practice or performed alone in a comfortable and steady position that eliminates any awareness of the physical body. Initially, deliberate conscious thought is necessary to direct the breath into a particular type of *pranayama*. Over time the awareness of the specific physical action of breathing moves into the subconscious background, substituted by a deepened state of meditative relaxation.

While exploring the posture sequences in a prior chapter, I suggested first settling into the foundational form of *pranayama, dirga pranayama,* or the complete yogic breath. We strive to maintain this deep diaphragmatic complete belly breath throughout our *asana* practice in order to connect the relaxing effects of the breath with the relaxing effects of a heightened awareness on the physical body and, when moving, the gentle waves of inhalation and exhalation with the ebb and flow of your unique flowing movements. As such, we are always integrating *pranayama* with our *asana* practice.

Pranayama is comprised of varying breathing techniques that differ in intensity and heat, ranging from energy channel activating techniques that fuel the *agni,* the inner fire, activate the energy of the sun and stir up deep-seated emotions, to energy channeling techniques, which cool the mind and body, activate the energy of the moon and allow one to become the objective witness to any uncovered emotions. A *pranayama* practice consists of a sequence of different breathing techniques designed to approximate a wave, one that progressively creates more and more psychic and physical heat, progressing from energy channelling to channel activating forms, until it ultimately crests, eventually subsiding with emotional and physical cooling and self-reflection. Similar to the practice of the *asanas, pranayama* takes time to master before it becomes emotionally impactful. Mastery is more easily realized through a dedication to a regular practice.

Both *pranayama* and the *asanas* represent two paths to access the spirit and create clarity of mind. They are complementary and both important to the practice of yoga. Typically in yoga, we attempt to connect inhalations to movements that open the body, physically facilitate deep, diaphragmatic breathing and spiritually promote the intake of *prana,* and exhalations to those that close the body, force air from the lungs and expel *apana,* or negative energy and mental waste. The sun breath is an excellent example of these receptive and expulsive actions. The sun breath begins with energizing the body from the ground up; grounding feet into the mat, activating the muscles of the legs and elongating the torso and spine. With a deep, diaphragmatic inhalation, arms are swept overhead and shoulders are pulled back to create a gentle backbend, thereby opening up the body. With a long exhalation, energy is released as you swan dive down into a standing, forward fold.

In his *Yoga Sutras,* felt to have been written sometime in the first millennium, Pantanjali defines *asana*, the third of the Eight Limbs of Yoga, as a position that is steady and comfortable in which to master *pranayama*, the fourth limb, before attempting to master the four subsequent limbs that represent deeper and deeper successive states of meditation. His system of yoga did not include the system of various postures that we practice today. And, although *pranayama* reflects a more ancient practice that antedates our modern day version of yoga, it has become a lost art in the Western world. Unfortunately, in most yoga classes, most, or even all of the emphasis is placed on the performance of the *asanas* at the expense of time in *pranayama*. If at all, a teacher may guide their class through a short round of *pranayama* at any point in a class, possibly two to five minutes, more often at the beginning, and less so at the end. At the beginning of the class, *pranayama* serves to center the class and allows for a transition from thoughts of the day to thoughts of one's practice. Centering is bringing oneself into the center of the room, into the center of self and into the moment. *Pranayama* is also a way to establish a deep, diaphragmatic breath before it is linked to movement, as well as to set the tone of relaxation for the remainder of the class. If performed near the end of a class, *pranayama* can serve as a bridge from physical activity to the quietude and relaxation of *shavasana*. Of course, as yoga need not be done in a class, one can certainly integrate *pranayama* into a personalized home practice.

Unlike the expression of the *asanas,* which differ from

person to person and are dependent on both acquired and genetically-based flexibility and strength, the practice of *pranayama* has a more level playing field. Except for people afflicted with pulmonary, muscular or neurological diseases, we all have a similar capacity to breathe. Spiritually, *pranayama* can balance and distribute *prana,* the life force, throughout the body. Physiologically, breathing is the mechanism whereby oxygen is brought into the body and carbon dioxide removed. Oxygen is also a life force. Without it, our cells would lose the ability to produce energy. Whether from yogic philosophical or physiological perspectives, optimizing and controlling the flow of breath nourishes the body with a life force.

With most forms of *pranayama,* breathing is done by inhaling and exhaling through the nose. Awareness of the breath is heightened by focusing on the sound, the feel of the breath or the physical actions of the body used to control the breath specific to each technique. Regardless of the type of breathing technique, any physical discomfort will flood the mind with negative sensations that will disrupt single-pointed focus on the breath. In positioning the body for *pranayama,* two conditions should be met. One is sitting without physical discomfort or strain. The other is sitting in a position that allows for the greatest downward excursion of the diaphragm with inhalation.

The diaphragm is a dome-shaped muscle that divides the chest from the abdomen. With inhalation it moves downward into the abdomen as it sucks air into the lungs. Limitations to maximizing breath control arise more so from incorrect posture than the ability to breathe. Rounding of the back "crunches" and crowds the abdominal contents, as the intestines and organs are pushed together. With less room in the abdomen, downward movement of the diaphragm is limited, resulting in a decrease in lung capacity. Elongation of the spine and relaxing the shoulders down the back affords more space in the abdomen, greater inferior diaphragmatic movement and a more optimal breath. Elongation of the spine is best accomplished by sitting on the edge of a cushion or bolster in order to bring the hips above the level of the knees, thereby lessening the tendency to round the back. Sitting in a chair or on two blocks while kneeling in a supported hero's pose are alternative, effective ways to elongate the spine and open up the abdomen. Once elongation of the spine and torso are achieved, the ability to perform *pranayama* transcends age and physical limitations.

As is true of performing the *asanas,* safety is paramount in the practice of *pranayama.* Precautions and contraindications exist, especially for the more vigorous and heat-producing forms, such as *anuloma viloma, kapalabhati,* and *bhastrika;* all more often done with breath retention. Contraindications, which are also mentioned in the appendix, include pregnancy, recent abdominal surgery, abdominal or pelvic hernias, glaucoma, uncontrolled hypertension and pulmonary and/or cardiovascular diseases, among many others. Some consider menstruation a precaution. Of course, nasal congestion and resistance to breathing due to a deviated septum could pose a problem. In the practice of yoga, as well as any other activity, consulting with a medical professional can be helpful if you possess any doubts regarding any medical condition that might represent a contraindication. It is also advised to have some proficiency at the less heat-activating types of *pranayama* before attempting the more vigorous forms that can be more emotionally charged and physically taxing.

Finally, approach the practice of *pranayama* with self-kindness and non-attachment to the goal of achieving meditative states. Simply consider it as as one of many ways to relax. Keep an open mind as you consider these techniques. They may prove to be valuable tools to help you cope. In addition, you can better choose those aspects of yoga that speak to you most if you experience all that it has to offer.

The following is an exploration of the many different forms of *pranayama*. You might decide to create a formal *pranayama* practice, integrate some of these techniques into your *asana* practice or choose one or two to perform to promote relaxation through meditation. As always, you are in the proverbial driver's seat with an exciting opportunity to create your own version of yoga.

Dirga Pranayama
The Three Part Complete Yogic Breath

The Sanskrit word *dirga* translates to "full" or "complete." Many consider this complete yogic breath the foundational breathing technique, as it serves to warm-up the muscles of respiration by progressively stretching them, as a normal breathing rhythm evolves into deep diaphragmatic breathing. *Dirga pranayama* also warms up the mind to be more receptive to new perspectives and self-discovery. *Dirga* breathing should become progressively deeper and longer with each inhalation and exhalation, until you are breathing into complete fullness and exhaling into complete emptiness. Once establishing full breathing capacity, other techniques, like *ujjayi* breathing and *nadi shodhana,* discussed below, can be added onto the frame-work of *dirga pranayama.*

Dirga pranayama is a three part breath. During inhalation, the three parts of the breath sequentially occur in the abdomen, the rib cage and the upper chest. The challenge is to add all three together into a single deep wave of motion. In order to learn this technique, however, it is useful to consider each part separately before combining them into a single, deep, complete breath. Resting one hand on the belly and one on the chest is useful in understanding the complete three part breath.

Part I ~ The Abdomen

After establishing a steady and comfortable seated position, begin by taking a deep inhalation to expand the belly alone. The lower hand resting on the belly is pushed out away from the body as you breathe in. Exhale out as much air as you can in order to draw the lower hand and belly button as close to the spine as possible. Take another deep inhalation allowing the belly to expand out like a balloon. Exhale to let the balloon collapse to complete emptiness.

Part II ~ The Ribcage

Now, inhale to expand the belly and let the breath travel up into the ribs as they flare out in all four directions. As you exhale completely, the ribs are drawn together and the belly collapses. Take another deep inhalation to first expand the belly and then the ribcage, imagining that the ribs are spreading apart like the gills of a fish, followed by a long exhalation.

Part III ~ The Upper Chest

Finally, inhale to expand the belly and let the breath travel up through the rib cage and all the way superiorly into the upper chest, causing the collar bones to lift up and out. Exhalation can occur in reverse from the upper chest to the lower belly.

An attempt should be made to make the exhalation longer than the inhalation, if possible. Take another deep inhalation and notice how the lower hand on the belly first moves away from the spine, and as the breath travels upward, the upper hand is then pushed out. Breath retention is considered a component of more advanced *pranayama,* but inserting a very short pause at the very top of the inhalation and the bottom of the exhalation can afford a few moments to appreciate stillness before reactivating the respiratory movements of the chest and abdomen.

Now the three parts of the breath can become one. Imagine the breath is a wave that spreads from the bottom of the belly all the way up to the collar bones. The wave pulls the belly from the spine, draws the ribs apart and then expands the chest. The wave ebbs and recedes during exhalation from the upper chest down to the lower belly. The full expression of *dirga pranayama* is realized by making smooth transitions between the three parts.

After establishing the rhythm of the breath, see if each breath can be slower and deeper than the one before. Let the gentle, yet full waves of breath become long. As the complete breath is established, attention can be brought not just to the sound of the breath, but also to the rhythm of the wave-like movements of the chest and abdomen. Eventually, as you fall into deeper meditative states you can be less deliberate in your observations.

Along with considering the complete yogic breath as a

vehicle for meditation and self-reflection, we can analyze what is occurring anatomically during the three parts of *dirga pranayama*.

- During the first part, expansion of the belly is caused by the downward excursion of the diaphragm as it displaces the moveable abdominal contents outward and downward. Inhalation occurs with a vacuum-like mechanism. One might imagine the downward pull of the diaphragm analogous to the inner stopper of a hypodermic syringe. As the stopper is pulled back, or in this case the diaphragm descending, air is sucked inside the lungs.
- During the second part, as air expands the lungs, the ribs are pushed outward and the intercostal muscles between the ribs are secondarily stretched.
- During the third part, air completely fills all of the air spaces of the lungs. The filling of the upper lobes of the lungs outwardly expands the upper chest and pushes the collar bones outward and upward.
- During exhalation, the intercostal muscles contract and pull the ribs together to actively push air out of the lungs. Concurrently, there is upward relaxation of the diaphragm.

Although an instructor may guide you through only a short period of *dirga pranayama*, ideally we wish to maintain long and deep diaphragmatic breathing throughout a class, which along with connecting it to our movements, is much more impactful in inducing relaxation and meditative states. And certainly, *dirga pranayama* need not be limited to a yoga class. It is a wonderful, meditative experience to enjoy at any time. Even just taking a few moments out of a hectic and stressful day to pause, close the eyes and take a deep, three part, diaphragmatic breath can relax the mind and reset the brain for the remainder of the day. Yoga is not just reserved for a class or studio.

Ujjayi Pranayama
The Victorious Breath

The *ujjayi* breath is also called the ocean sounding breath. It is created by breathing in and out of the nose while partially constricting the muscles in the back of the throat surrounding the glottis, the site of the vocal cords. It can be experienced by bringing your palm up close to your open mouth as you exhale, as if you are fogging up a mirror or cleaning your eyeglasses. This will create a "hah" sound and a sensation of warmth on your palm. That "hah" sound is a result of the constriction of the throat. Now, see if you can replicate that sound with inhalation. Once you feel comfortable with this breath, close your mouth and breathe through the nose while continuing to constrict the muscles of the throat. You will notice that the breath sounds like the waves of the ocean coming in to shore and back out to sea with each inhalation and exhalation. Once you have settled into the relaxing sounds of the ocean waves, see if you can increase the forcefulness of the breath. The resultant increase in sound volume facilitates single-pointed concentration.

The *ujjayi* breath can be layered upon *dirga pranayama*. In this regard, *dirga pranayama* is first established before adding the *ujjayi* breath. Several rounds of *dirga pranayama* begin to draw you inward. As the *ujjayi* breath is added, that inward force increases as you sink deeper into relaxation. In many yogic traditions, such as Ashtanga yoga, *ujjayi* breathing is done throughout a practice, although this is not exclusive to just this tradition. Regardless of the particular yoga practiced, the increased and peaceful sound of the breath becomes a constant reminder to connect your breath to your movements.

The Sanskrit word, "*ujjayi*" translates to victorious. How one's yoga practice is a victory is up to each one of us to determine. If the relaxing effects of *ujjayi pranayama* help you better face the challenges of life, then it is truly a victory.

Nadi Shodhana

Alternate Nostril Breathing or the Channel Clearing Breath

As previously discussed, the *nadis* are considered to be an extensive network of energy channels through which *prana,* the life force, flows throughout the body. Many of the *nadis* directly connect to the *chakras,* the seven main energy centers. *Nadi shodhana* is a yogic breathing technique designed to clear these energy channels, allowing for optimal flow and balance of *prana* throughout the body. Metaphorically, one might imagine the *nadis* clogged or obstructed by negative energy arising from thoughts that don't serve us at the present moment. *Nadi shodhana* is a practice of mindfulness that clears those obstructions to allow for the flow of positive ideas and emotions.

For *nadi shodhana,* the focus can be on the sound of the breath. Alternatively, focus can be on the rhythm of the hand and finger movements successively opening and closing the nostrils. The sound of the breath is the primary point of focus for all of the yogic breathing techniques, but what makes each form of *pranayama* unique is the actions of the physical body used to capture and control the breath.

As with all forms of meditation, starting in a comfortable and steady position is paramount. Traditionally, *nadi shodhana* is performed with the right hand in *Vishnu mudra*. In yogic philosophy, the right hand is symbolic of receptivity. Further-more, *Vishnu* is a Hindu deity known as the Preserver, who maintains the order in the universe, and on a personal level, hopefully some order in our thoughts. *Vishnu mudra* is created by bending the index and third fingers inward towards the palm. The extended ring finger is placed adjacent to the left nostril and the thumb next to the right. Begin by inhaling through both nostrils. Next, occlude the right nostril with the thumb as you exhale through the left. Then, inhale up the left nostril, open up the right, occlude the left with your ring finger and exhale through the right. Inhale up the right, occlude the right and exhale once again through the left. Breathing continues as such, alternating from nostril to nostril.

Once you have established the alternating rhythm between nostrils, begin to slow and deepen the breath to layer on *dirga pranayama*. You can then add *ujjayi* breathing, again to increase the sound volume of the breath and create the relaxing sounds of the ocean waves. Feelings of inwardness are deepened by bringing awareness to the sound of the breath, as well as to the rhythm of the fingers moving back and forth to occlude and release alternate nostrils.

As is true in life, in performing all of the *asanas* and *pranayama* in yoga, there are no hard and fast rules. This is equally true for *nadi shodhana*. As such, modifications are welcome. The *Vishnu mudra* is uncomfortable for some. The sustained flexion of the second and third fingers toward the palm requires continued contraction of the flexor muscles in the forearm, which can lead to muscle fatigue and discomfort. A modification that releases the engagement of the flexors involves extending the index and third fingers to rest on the forehead at the third eye center. You can also use the left hand and arm to support the right elbow if the right arm becomes fatigued. You can even do a hands-free version of *nadi shodhana*. Hands-free does not refer to using bluetooth, but rather imagining the breath flowing up one nostril and out through the other. Taking it one step further, one might imagine energy flowing from the foot to the crown of head on one side of the body with inhalation and energy flowing in the opposite direction down the other side of the body with exhalation. The focus becomes the long lines of energy flow that alternate from one side of the body to the other.

As mentioned, typically in a yoga class, time does not allow for an extended period of *pranayama. Nadi shodhana* is much more impactful and powerful as a meditative tool when performed over a prolonged period of time. It can be a wonderful part of a meditative practice done at home. The focus on the rhythms that you create can be hypnotic.

Nadi shodhana clears all of the energy channels, including the *sushumna nadi*, the main central energy channel that connects the *chakras* and carries the *kundalini* energy from the pelvis to crown of head. Clearing the other two main energy channels, the *ida* and *pingala nadis,* or the lunar and solar energy channels, facilitates the creation of a balance between the two. It is through this balance between the moon and the sun, rest and activity, heat and cooling, receptivity and irrationality, and the feminine and masculine selves that allows for the barriers to self-discovery, realization and personal growth to dissolve.

Anuloma Viloma
Alternate Nostril Breathing with Breath Retention

Anuloma viloma translates to "with the hair or grain and against the hair or grain". Imagine grooming a horse. Brushing the horse against the grain of its hair causes dirt, shedded skin and other particulate matter to be jarred loose from the horse's body. Brushing with the grain eliminates the resultant mess and smooths out the horse's coat.

Just like brushing against the grain, *anuloma viloma* stirs up emotions and past traumas. Like brushing with the grain, one can bear witness to what has been uncovered in order to smooth out the lasting effects of negative life experiences that press down upon the spirit.

Anuloma viloma is performed similar to *nadi shodhana,* but with the addition of a *kumbhaka,* or breath retention, of variable length. If the breath is held at the top of inhalation it is called the inner or *antar kumbhaka* and at the end of exhalation, the outer or *bahya kumbhaka.* The longer the breath is held, the more heat is produced and the more emotionally-activating the *pranayama* becomes.

The uncovering and witnessing of repressed emotions and trauma that comes with the more vigorous, heat-producing *pranayama,* especially those that employ a *kumbhaka,* may not initially be accessible. Just like a practice of the *asanas,* gradual realization of the benefits of a regular *pranayama* practice takes time and patience. *Anuloma viloma* is considered a more advanced practice and should be reserved only after the more basic, less activating forms of *pranayama* are mastered. Unlike *dirga, ujjayi* and *nadi shodhana* breathing, which are relatively safe with few precautions, the contraindications mentioned above and listed in the appendix exist any time a *kumbhaka* is used. The outer or *bahya kumbhaka* is considered more strenuous, heat-producing and emotionally impactful than the inner or *antar kumbhaka* since holding one's breath at the end of exhalation, when one is depleted of oxygen, is much more difficult. Of course, the longer the breath is held, the more vigorous your experience. At its extreme, a breath retention causes the body to hunger for air that can translate into a hunger for the resolution of past traumas and disturbing emotions with the potential for subsequent peace of mind.

Kapalabhati Pranayama

The Skull Shining Breath or The Breath of Fire

Kapalabhati is a Sanskrit compound word made up of *kapal* meaning "skull" and *bhati* meaning "shining" or "enlightening". *Kapalabhati pranayama* is a purification technique, directed at clearing the cranial paranasal sinuses of mucus and secretions. Spiritually, its explosive quality activates and energizes the body and mind, stirring up repressed emotions and past traumas felt to be held deep in the pelvis. It awakens the *kundalini,* depicted as a coiled snake at the base of spine. It's the divine feminine energy, that once activated, travels up the spine in the process of spiritual liberation. Once thoughts and feelings of past experiences are revealed through the physical and emotional power of *kapalabhati pranayama,* the opportunity exists to bear witness to once hidden emotions with the hope of understanding them and disarming their power.

To learn *kapalabhati* breathing, place both hands, stacked one on top of the other, on the upper belly. Both the inhalations and exhalations occur quickly and at a rapid pace. The exhalation is a short, powerful burst created by forceful contraction of the abdominal muscles, actively and quickly pulling them toward the spine. The inhalation occurs passively, as the abdominal muscles release, thereby rapidly sucking air into the lungs. In short bursts, the contraction and release of the abdominal muscles will cause the stacked hands to move quickly and sharply toward and away from the spine during exhalation and inhalation. Once you become accustomed to this action, you can release the hands down to the thighs or lap. Frequency of the inhalations and exhalations and duration of *kapalabhati* breathing varies from practitioner to practitioner. One example of the frequency of the breathing cycle that might be used is one to two breaths per second for eight to ten cycles. Often, continued *kapalabhati* breathing will begin to clear mucus and secretions from the nose and sinuses, so it is a good idea to have a tissue nearby.

There are many contraindications to the performance of *kapalabhati pranayama,* many of which again are mentioned above and listed in the appendix. It bears noting that this rapid type of breathing in short bursts can lead to hypoventilation with symptoms of lightheadedness and dizziness. As such, it should not be practiced by individuals with high or low blood pressure, heart disease, or history of prior stroke. Of course, if you experience lightheadedness, stop *kapalabhati* immediately and return back to the deep, full breaths of *dirga pranayama.*

Depression and anxiety often deplete energy. The inherent vigor of *kapalabhati pranayama* can also deplete energy, but in a beneficial way, by releasing physical and mental tension.

Bhastrika Pranayama
Bellows Breath

Bhastrika is also considered a vigorous, heat producing type of *pranayama*, but even more so than *kapalabhati*. As such, it should be reserved for those that have an established *pranayama* practice. It is done similar to *kapalabhati,* but instead of forced exhalations and passive inhalations, both exhalations and inhalations are actively and forcibly performed. Similar contraindications and precautions exist for *bhastrika* as with *kapalabhati.*

Bandhas
Locks

Both *bhastrika* and *kapalabhati* are often done in conjunction with locks or *bandhas,* the sustained contraction of specific regional muscle groups. The *bandhas* are typically performed with breath retention, or *kumbhaka.*

There are three commonly used *bandhas:*

1. *Mula bandha mudra,* or the root lock. This lock involves the sustained contraction of the perineal muscles, similar to a Kegel exercise.
2. *Uddiyana bandha mudra,* or the stomach lock. This is done exclusively during breath retention after exhalation and involves contracting the abdominal muscles and pulling them up under the ribs.
3. *Jalandhara bandha mudra* or the throat lock, a contraction of the muscles of the larynx. One performs this lock by sustaining a half swallow.

Bhastrika and *kapalabhati* can also be followed by *agni sara,* an undulation of the abdominal muscles done with an outer *kumbhaka. Agni sara* translates to "the essence of fire". *Agni* is the fire that burns deep in the belly. It might be considered a metaphor for one's zest and enthusiasm for life.

A proviso for these emotionally impactful breathing techniques is to proceed with caution. With the intention of self-analysis, revisiting prior traumas might be too disturbing and uncomfortable to bear. That analysis might be easier and more gentle with other types of therapy, including those done with a professional trained in psychotherapy.

Sitali Pranayama

The Cooling Breath

As opposed to *pranayama* techniques like *kapalabhati* and *bhastrika,* which are channel activating, energizing and heat-producing, *sitali pranayama* is cooling and energy channeling. *Kapalabhati* and *bhastrika* can stir up emotions deep in the pelvis, activating the energy of the sun. By then performing *sitali,* energy is channeled to the moon pathway, allowing the more rational self to bear witness to feelings and thoughts. This process can dissolve *anhankara,* the perceived self that often can be illusory, and thereby revealing one's true authenticate self.

Sitali is the most cooling of all of the *pranayama* techniques and is appropriate after the wave of heat crests from the aforementioned channel activating breaths. To perform *sitali,* exhale out fully through the nose to complete emptiness. Stick a curled tongue out between the lips and inhale slowly through the tube that is formed. You will experience a cooling sensation on the tongue and in the mouth. When you have inhaled completely, hold your breath for a moment and lightly touch the tip of your tongue to the roof of your mouth, either on the hard or soft palate, as far back as possible without causing discomfort on the undersurface of the tongue and frenulum, the connection of the tongue to the midline of the floor of the oral cavity. You can revert to a normal breathing rhythm or do a short round of *dirga pranayama* before returning back to the *sitali* breath. The light touch of the cool tip of the tongue on the palate becomes a single point of focus around which self-reflection occurs.

Sitkari Pranayama
The Hissing Breath

The Sanskrit word *sitkari* translates to "hissing". *Sitkari* is the alternative to *sitali* for those that are unable to curl their tongues; approximately one quarter to one third of the population. *Sitkari* is performed the same as *sitali* except that the tongue remains in the mouth. The tip of the tongue is lightly touched to where the upper and lower teeth meet. Typically, the jaw is opened to separate the teeth ever so slightly. As inhalation occurs, the tongue approximates a shallow bowl shape. At the top of inhalation, the tip of the tongue is again touched to the palate to serve as your point of focus. Similar to *sitali, sitkari* cools the tongue and mouth. Note that *sitkari* may be uncomfortable for those with sensitive teeth.

Bhramari Pranayama
Female Bee Breath

Bhramari is also a cooling, energy channeling breath, often done after a round or rounds of channel activating *kapalabhati* and/or *bhastrika*. *Bhramari* is the Hindu Goddess of the Black Bees. During exhalation, a humming sound is created, emulating the sound of a bee. The tip of the tongue is first firmly pressed up against the hard palate as one inhales fully. Upon exhaling, humming is done through the nose and throat. Since this is the female bee breath, traditionally one creates a high pitch sound. One can experiment, however, with lower frequencies and observe how that changes your experience.

Bhramari is often done in conjunction with *yoni mudra*. The Sanskrit word *yoni* means "womb." *Yoni mudra* is dedicated to Shakti, the goddess that is responsible for creation and who represents the divine, feminine, cosmic energy in the universe. *Yoni mudra* simulates a detachment from the world with a quieting of the mind similar to a fetus in the womb. As such, the hand position is directed at blocking out all experience of external stimuli. With both hands brought up toward the face, the second and third fingers are lightly placed over the eyelids, symbolic of the elimination of the sense of vision. The fourth fingers are placed under the nose, symbolic of the elimination of the sense of smell. Pinky fingers lie just under the mouth, within which is the sense of taste. The thumbs are then used to press the tragus of each ear, a small flap of cartilage protruding from each ear just in front of the external ear canal, to occlude the ear canals. Occluding the ear canals intensifies the sound of the bee as it fills the head with its vibratory energy. Focusing on that sound can be quite meditative and, as such, a longer period of sustained bee breath can be more beneficial for stress reduction.

Simhasana Pranayama
Lion's Breath

The Lion's Breath is done while in *simhasana,* the lion's pose. There are several ways to enter into the lion's pose. One can begin in the hero's pose. The palms are then placed face down in front of the knees, fingers either pointed towards or away from the body, as the torso leans forward. Variations include sitting on curled toes or bringing the inner edges of the feet to touch, knees out wide. Once in *simhasana,* one then sticks the tongue out from the mouth and, with a strong exhalation, lets out a loud roar, the roar of the lion. The forcefulness of the lion's breath is felt to be beneficial to release anger. Creating this breath, especially in unison with a room full of fellow classmates, can also be quite a humorous experience, which even more so helps to dissolve any negative feelings. Yoga need not always be a serious pursuit. A bit of humor and laughter can go a long way to reduce stress.

A *Pranayama* Practice

A *pranayama* practice is the creation of a sequence of the various forms of *pranayama*. Similar to posture sequences to de-stress, a sequence of the differing forms of yogic breathing techniques can have profound, relaxing effects. Deliberate single-pointed concentration is needed to master the various aspects that define each technique. As mentioned previously, it is advised to have some proficiency at the less heat-activating types of *pranayama* before attempting the more vigorous forms that can be more emotionally charged.

A *pranayama* practice is constructed like a wave. The wave begins to form with *dirga pranayama* and *ujjayi* breathing that serve to warm up the muscles of respiration and begin to fuel the fire of emotions. The wave crests with the performance of the channel activating, heat producing forms of *pranayama*, such as *anuloma viloma*, *kapalabhati* and *bhastrika*. Heat is intensified by adding *kumbhakas, bandhas* and *agni sara*. Progressive cooling then occurs as the wave subsides, fueling the lunar energy and allowing for self-reflection. A cooling sequence might consist of *nadi shodhana, brahmari,* and *sitali* or *sitkari*.

Many variations for sequencing *pranayama* exist, all for the most part following a similar warmup-heat-cooling waveform. Easing slowly into a *pranayama* practice is important. Starting with a lesser number of rounds of the more heat producing forms of *pranayama* will ultimately prove to be more beneficial than jumping right into the heat. The use of *kumbhakas, bandhas* and *agni sara* should be reserved for more advanced practitioners. Progress occurs gradually. Patience is paramount.

Whether or not you commit to a regular, dedicated *pranayama* practice, it is still worthwhile to experiment with these different techniques of yogic breathing. It will give you a better appreciation for the practice of the ancient yogis. Since *pranayama* is completely breath-focused, trying it will also help you to be more cognizant of your breath when performing the *asanas*. Familiarity with *pranayama* can also help you integrate the breath with your movements.

As with yoga and life, realistic expectations are paramount. Attachment to future outcomes, including the possibility of a life-changing epiphany, will set you up to fail. Regardless of whether or not these breathing techniques are emotionally impactful, single-pointed concentration on the breath and the physical action of the body that define each type of *pranayama* can induce deep states of relaxation. Learning these techniques is learning to relax.

Pranayama can become one more tool to calm an active

mind and any rumination on disturbing thoughts. It is through learned relaxation that the ill-effects of depression and anxiety become less onerous. Quite simply, we breathe into our yoga, and through dedication to its practice, we learn to breathe into relaxation.

13

CALMING THE STORM

Perhaps as an author, I am guilty of an overuse of metaphors. However, they can serve as useful constructs to apply common ideas to experiences that are often beyond description. So I will take the liberty to use "a storm" as a metaphor for an acute episode of depression or anxiety. There are many different types of storms. Like a tornado, an acute episode can occur without warning, wreaking havoc along its path. Like a hurricane, acute depression and anxiety can be overwhelming, flooding the mind with inescapable pain. Like a blizzard, they can bury you deep in despair, immobilized by disturbing thoughts and emotions that potentially lead to self-harm. An unrealistic expectation might be held that when the storm finally abates a rainbow will appear and everything will be alright. Rather, our hope is to calm the storm as much as possible in hopes of transitioning into a safe space. Once there is a break from the maelstrom of unrelenting negative thoughts and images that plague the mind during a crisis, working toward achieving a modicum of peace can be reinitiated.

As it always bears repeating, it is paramount to reach out for support if an acute episode of depression or anxiety is unmanageable with thoughts of self-harm, whether it be to a professional, family member, friend, or hotline. Even if one doesn't harbor thoughts of self-harm, an acute episode can nonetheless be fraught with often unbearable psychic pain that is worsened when experienced alone.

Restrained by an overwhelming flood of negative thoughts, one can be left devoid of energy and mired in hopelessness for any relief from the psychic pain that weighs down upon the spirit like a vague force holding one under the water. Occupied by a need to just survive, self-care is not a priority. How then does one find the wherewithal to access the benefits of yoga? Can yoga be expected to bring one to a better place while in crisis?

As discussed, learned relaxation through yoga includes establishing a single point of focus through mindfulness of physical sensations or novel thoughts and ideas. I might argue that one does possess single-pointed focus while suffering through an episode of deep depression or acute anxiety, but unfortunately the object of focus is a disturbing thought or thoughts that don't serve in the moment. Even more so, the point of focus is a destructive one. Rumination on suffering can be all-consuming. The workings of the mind are usurped by a heightened awareness of unrelenting inner pain and hopelessness.

Often in yoga, our goal is to connect to one's inner self to gain insight and awareness of true passions and desires. Perhaps, it is best not to delve deeply into the content of disturbing thoughts during an acute episode of depression or anxiety, but rather, and arguably much more beneficial to "get out of one's head", to divert attention away from the inner self.

Most everything we attempt in life is easier said than done, however, redirecting thoughts away from inner turmoil to an object of focus external to the self may possess the power to refocus the brain away from the storm of painful thoughts. This might be as simple as taking a deep breath and noticing the sound you create. When stressed, we often take shallow breaths. Deep breathing brings the parasympathetic and sympathetic responses into balance. The despair inherent to an acute depressive episode or the waves of tension and unease that crash and wash over the mind in a panic attack or other acute episode of anxiety can become less onerous by redirecting thought to deep breathing and, more specifically, to the sound of the breath. Although you are the one breathing, the sound that you make exists outside of yourself. The sound you hear represents the expansion and compression of air molecules external to the body resulting from your inhalations and exhalations.

Since during a depressive episode or a period of acute anxiety psychic pain emanates from an uncomfortable mind, I believe it is not practical to battle with disturbing thoughts by attempting to replace them with more positive ones. Being told to think of something pleasant or to cheer up isn't very effective in calming the mind. Once again, what carries a greater potential in that regard is focusing on a sensation produced by the experience of something external to the mind. Breathing into a physical sensation may be even more effective than simply listening to the breath in order to refocus the mind away from inner turmoil.

In order to redirect attention away from disturbing thoughts, we can use our senses. Each breath taken into each sensation you experience is one step closer to diverting attention away from hopelessness and despair. Perhaps, you can do a body scan, noticing touch sensations.

In that regard, you can try an exercise right now. Assuming that you are sitting as you read,

- first draw your attention to the feeling of your feet on the floor, noticing the contact points of each toe
- next bring your focus to the feeling of the back of each thigh on the chair
- then notice the sensation resulting from the touch of the fabric of your shirt on your body

- next notice where your fingers are positioned and what they are touching. Explore what is touching each fingertip and if one differs from the other
- next turn your attention to the touch of the fabric of your pants and socks on each leg

During this exercise, where were your thoughts? Hopefully, they were directed to the sensations of touch. A mindfulness scan can be very effective in "getting out of one's head" and redirecting the internal self to the experience of the external world. For the sense of touch, what is contacting the body exists external to the body. This exercise is even more impactful if you breathe deeply into each touch sensation. This gives you a so-called "two for one" bargain; the relaxing effects of a deep breath are layered upon those emanating from a mindfulness body scan.

Alternatively, you might explore the sense of proprioception with eyes closed and breathe deeply into the position of outstretched arms and legs in space, the awareness of which comes from the body sensing the effects of gravity on each limb. Through aromatherapy, breathing into a pleasing scent, maybe emanating from essential oils in a diffuser, can also have a calming effect. Once again, breathing deeply into a sensation caused by the experience of something external to yourself may be enough to pull you away from the internal self, even if it is only partially effective or momentary. In acute episodes of depression and anxiety, any relief is welcomed no matter how fleeting.

Consider two people. Both are in crisis. Their psychic pain is unbearable. Questions of life's meaning arise. Perhaps, both people are hyper-focused on the hopelessness of their situations; a feeling that there is no relief from the mental pain caused by their disease. Person one continues to ruminate. By remaining focused on their hopeless situation there is a limited potential to defuse the crisis. The other person, person two, takes a deep breath that starts from the belly and spreads upward to expand the upper chest followed by a slower exhalation, what we call *dirga pranayama,* the complete yogic breath. For just a very short moment, rumination is interrupted by an awareness of the sound of a deep breath and the comforting stretch of the belly and chest. By continuing to breathe deeply and listening to each inhalation and exhalation entering and exiting the nose, a series of interruptions of thought are linked together. Attention shifts to the breath. Now, person two chooses to scan the body and deeply breathe into any touch sensations affecting each body part or noticing the position of parts of the body in space. Although potentially fleeting, thoughts are once again diverted away from the deep dark place of the mind to the external world, increasing the likelihood that person two will emerge from crisis.

Sometimes implementing the aforementioned process is facilitated by someone else, possibly a friend, family member or other support person guiding the person in crisis through a mindfulness exercise. Often those whom are in a supportive role feel powerless to help. Guiding someone through a mindfulness exercise is a practical method to help someone in a nonjudgmental way.

With the aforementioned said, the reality is that for those that suffer, redirecting disturbing, inner thought patterns to what is occurring in the external world can be a herculean effort. If successful, however, thoughts of hopelessness, pain and despair that possess so much destructive power can be replaced by thoughts of objective observations that possess no emotional power. Initial and then repeated success at this process can increase its effectiveness in the future.

Once the storm of acute depression or anxiety has abated, self-care and a return to the sanctity of your full yoga practice can be reinitiated. It is always paramount to treat yourself with self-kindness. So don't beat yourself up for succumbing to the storm in the first place. We can only try our best in life. Be proud of any attempt to be your best. Realize that despite your misperceptions of weakness and failure, you are someone with inner strength. Inherent to these debilitating diseases is a persistent feeling of weakness of character. Experiencing opposites in life often gives us a better sense of each one than experienced separately. Perhaps, experiencing what is perceived as a weakness of character can allow you to know your inner strength that much more. Be proud of taking action to help yourself by reading this book. Let your yoga be a practice that both strengthens the body and mind.

Throughout this book, I have presented a lot of information to digest, as my intention has been to offer you different paths that lead to the same goal of learned relaxation. I applaud you if you have stuck with me to this point. So now would be a good time to take a moment, simply pause, close your eyes, take a well-deserved deep belly breath and slowly exhale to complete relaxation. I think I'll do the same!

14

THE CODA

I possess a great love for music. I often look at a yoga class in musical terms. Like a symphony, there are changing dynamics, flowing themes and changes in mood and emotions. Most classical symphonies end with a coda, the final concluding musical passage. The coda is the last chance for a composer to impact the listener emotionally, as the themes of the opus come to a meaningful conclusion. Similarly, the very end of a yoga class is the last opportunity the instructor has to leave his, her or their students with a profound idea that connects the practice of yoga with living a meaningful life. The composer writes with the hope of inducing an emotional change in the listener, no matter how fleeting it might be. The yoga instructor has a similar hope by imparting thoughtful words to the student. For myself, my final words are not primarily directed at those in my class, but mainly toward myself. I choose to expose my own thoughts, emotions, wishes and ideals. They may resonate with some and not with others. I often speak of finding one's true authentic self, not living life with an expectation of what you think someone else wants you to be. I speak of practicing self-kindness with the hope of having compassion for others. I speak of tapping into one's inner strength with a positive perspective to better face life's challenges.

One does not need to practice yoga to experience any revelations. Yoga is merely a vehicle that facilitates the process. My yoga practice allows me to be introspective and gain insight. In an attempt to be an authentic teacher and not a version of what I think my students wish me to be, I end my classes with my own words that come deep from my heart and reflect who I am and the principles by which I live.

Classical symphonies are written in a particular key. Minor keys tend to be darker in mood, solemn and can possess a certain sadness. Major keys tend to be more joyful, filling the music with hope and promise. Often composers create an interplay between minor and major keys in order to present varying moods throughout their music. Often, minor and major keys seem to be in a grand battle; misery and suffering at odds with the triumph of the human spirit. It is my hope that as you arrive at this coda, you have learned to better access the major keys of life with new perspectives that can help you experience the triumph of hope and joy over pain and despair.

I often view my own life in terms of minor and major keys.

Life is a struggle, but through my practice of yoga I am spending less time in pain and despair and more with hope for peace and contentment. My goal is that through my life's work, the major key will win out over the minor. I wish to turn a negative into a positive; years of suffering and pain from mental illness transformed into something useful and tangible to help others. In a sense, the negative was necessary to discover the positive. Similar to a better appreciation of the warmth of a house when coming in from the frigid cold, by knowing the pain and suffering inherent to depression and anxiety, I am better able to appreciate the opposite extreme of contentment and peace. That then allows me to possess greater empathy for others. That ability has been enhanced through my practice of yoga, with a dedication to kindness and compassion. My battle with life-long depression and anxiety has created a frame of reference that allows me to gain meaning and satisfaction that much more. I can be grateful for the marvels of the world that surround me when I am in a less depressed state or during a period of relative normalcy. Of course, the times during which I can achieve feelings of deep gratitude may be short-lived and fleeting, but when they occur, they represent the richness of life that lets my spirit soar. I look at those times every time as a blessing. When I am depressed, I lose the ability to cry, as my depression is not sadness, but rather a muting of emotions. When I am able to connect to the beauty of life, my tears are those of joy.

My journey into yoga has lead me to a better appreciation

for the best parts of life. I have undergone a personal transformation with a life full of newfound hope. I realized that chronic depression and anxiety usurped my ability to appreciate the gifts that I was given.

Realistic expectations are critical when approaching any facet of life. As it bears repeating, yoga is not a cure for mental illness, but an effective tool that complements other therapies. Based on suffering from a life-long illness, my expectation is that I will always have chronic depression and anxiety, but I am comforted by my newfound knowledge that by harnessing the power of yoga I can better cope and gain a deeper appreciation for all of life's blessings.

We all possess an inner beauty that is accessed by peeling away all of the layers of ugliness that is inherent to mental disease. One must not let mental disease define you. Depression and anxiety are what you have and not who you are. Perhaps like myself, however, it is difficult to separate the symptoms from your belief system. As such, inherent to your mental disease may be a limited ability to like yourself. Through yoga, however, it is worth the attempt to discover if a revelation can occur that deep in your spirit lies a unique, beautiful person, worthy of love and respect.

At the beginning of my yoga teacher training at Kripalu, we were asked to write our intention for being there on a particular shape made of colored construction paper that would hang on the walls of the classroom for the entire program. My intention was, and continues to be, "To help others with gratitude." I am truly grateful to have the opportunity to offer you the gift of yoga. It is a true privilege I have been given.

Finally, I hope that my words will ease your pain and help you better cope with the challenges that you face. Overcoming them can provide you with the gift of newfound pride, inner strength and hope. Embrace yoga and you will open up to limitless new perspectives that can enrich your life. Remember to practice in the context of realistic expectations. Try not to attach to final outcomes, especially finding a cure for what you suffer. Rather, enjoy the process, have pride in making the attempt and savor even the smallest of successes. Change happens gradually and requires patience. By choosing to read this book, you have already taken a step towards changing your perspective and, in the process, hopefully discovered that you do have some control over what you thought you never had.

Gratitude is the prerequisite for all other positive emotions that we experience. Gratitude enables one to develop a clear perspective of what is truly important in life. And when you have gratitude, you can have love and compassion. When you have love and compassion, the world will be yours, and the light within you and the light that is you will burn so brightly for everyone to see!

As I always close my yoga classes with words from my heart, perhaps it is most fitting to close this book by connecting to words from your heart. To that end, enter into a quiet space and find a comfortable and steady position in which to sit. Establish a deep breath with inhalations that spread like peaceful waves from the bottom of the belly to the top of the chest and with longer exhalations that spread downward. Concentrate on the sound of the breath going in and out of the nose. Once you have settled into this meditative breath, deeply inhale both arms overhead and bring the palms together in *anjali mudra,* or prayer hands. Inhale deeply once again. With your next exhalation, allow the hands to descend weightlessly to the forehead, the site of the *anja chakra*, or third eye *chakra*, the energy center for insight. With pride in yourself and your willingness to take on whatever challenges you face, take several deep breaths into an awareness of the unique person that you are. When you are ready, take another deep inhalation and upon exhalation, allow the hands to now float down to the heart center, the site of the *anahata chakra*, the energy center for love and compassion; in yogic philosophy assigned a green color. Bring to mind a picture of someone for whom you are grateful. Inhale deeply into those feelings of gratitude. Continue to breathe deeply. Imagine the green color of the *anahata chakra* as a warming, comforting light, the energy of your gratitude, glowing brighter and brighter with each inhalation. As you find deeper and deeper breaths, the energy intensifies to a point where the soothing, beautiful green light of gratitude begins to spread from your heart center throughout the rest of your body. With each breath, experience this manifestation of love spread from the chest, down the arms to the fingertips, into the torso and down the legs to the toes. Finally, allow the energy of your gratitude to fill your entire mind, leaving no room for any other thought. And now, with your body and mind completely aglow with the energy of gratitude, look deeply into your heart and find words of gratitude for yourself and all the blessings of your life!

Namaste!

> *The light that is within me honors and bows to the light within you. May your light shine brightly with all the love and compassion in your heart!*

Shanti, Shanti, Shanti!

> *May you find peace!*

Jai Bhagwan!

> *May your life be a blessed victory! May that victory let your spirit soar!*

AFTERWORD

While writing this book, my yellow lab, Bella, passed away. I recognize that death is part of the circle of life and that dogs unfortunately have a limited life span, but nonetheless grief was unavoidable. She was a grounding force in my life. In a sense, she was my therapy dog. Although she couldn't communicate with words, I could always feel her caring presence and love. She could sense when I was depressed and suffering in pain. Her expressions of unconditional love grounded me and got me through the most difficult of times.

I thought it was apropos that I should dedicate a book about coping with mental illness in her memory. She taught me that life is worth living and meaning lay in the love and support of others.

As an author, I always try to write from my heart with gratitude. I am grateful that I had her in my life. She taught me that gratitude brings happiness.

And for anyone who is faced with the challenges of mental illness, "happiness" is the most precious of words!

APPENDIX

Contraindications to the Asanas and Pranayama

It is paramount that yoga is practiced with an awareness of one's physical limitations in order prevent injury or a worsening of pre-existing disease states. In that regard, I will present a general list of the more common contraindications to the practice of the *asanas,* the poses, and *pranayama,* the yogic breathing techniques. As noted in the introduction, contradictions are medical conditions that disqualify someone from doing a particular activity. This is not a comprehensive list, so if you have any question or concern regarding any medical condition or injury you may have, consult your physician or other health professional for a definitive answer that will assure your health and wellbeing.

There are relative and absolute contraindications to the practice of yoga. A relative contraindication is one where conditions may or may not exist that could result in physical harm. For example, shoulder arthritis is a relative contraindication to assuming a high plank, where undue stress may be put on the shoulder girdle. Whether or not it is wise to assume a high plank is dependent on the individual practitioner and the extent of their injury or condition. A yoga instructor or author cannot realistically know the extent or seriousness of your injury or disease to pass judgment if something is safe or not. As such, all physical injuries are relative contraindications, since the decision to enter into an *asana* or a type of *pranayama* is up to the individual, hopefully based on complete knowledge of the extent of their injury from a prior diagnostic evaluation. One must always listen to the body to ensure that any pre-existing acute or chronic injury is not exacerbated by any movement or position. An unrealistic expectation is that yoga is beneficial for any malady. Yoga certainly possesses a host of benefits, but it should be practiced in the context of its potential detriment to any physical ailment, along with an acute awareness of the physical body.

Absolute contraindications are conditions that preclude one from assuming an *asana* or performing *pranayama* under any condition without exception. In fact, your physician or other health professional might have the opinion that certain diseases are absolute contraindications to doing yoga at all. They will also be able to help you distinguish whether a contraindication is absolute or relative. Please value their opinion. Important to the practice of yoga is creating a safe space, both mentally and physically. It requires having a deep understanding of your mind and body. To that end, it is often a trained health professional that can best guide you toward that understanding.

Contraindications
Asanas

- Uncontrolled high or low blood pressure
- Pregnancy (especially after the first trimester), especially prone postures, anything that

compresses the abdomen or extreme twisting postures

- Acute or chronic back, neck, abdominal pain and/or injury
- Recent abdominal or pelvic surgery
- Hernias, including inguinal and abdominal
- Ear or eye inflammation, injury or disease, especially for inversion postures where the heart is above the head.
- Sinus infection, especially for inversions
- Glaucoma, especially for inversions
- Dizziness, vertigo
- Shoulder, wrist, hip, knee, ankle and spinal injuries and conditions
- Menstrual abdominal cramps may worsen, especially with inversions
- Muscle tightness and injury, especially hamstrings and achilles tendon
- Abdominal discomfort due to digestive diseases
- Any emotional triggers

Pranayama

- Throat inflammation
- Sinus disease
- Dizziness, vertigo
- Uncontrolled hypetension

- Recent abdominal or pelvic surgery
- Epilepsy
- Nasal disease and congestion
- Menstrual abdominal cramps may worsen, especially with *kapalabhati* and *bhastrika*
- Abdominal discomfort due to digestive diseases
- Any emotional triggers

Once again, the aforementioned lists are not meant to be comprehensive, but represent some of the more common contraindications. Any questions regarding conditions that are not included on these lists and a more complete exploration of the specific implications of any disease entity in the context of a yoga practice are best addressed with your health care professional. Always proceed conservatively with caution to honor your body. And of course in the context of the themes of this book, always practice yoga with a connection to thoughts and emotions to be able to fully honor the mind.

ABOUT THE AUTHOR

Gordon Kanzer discovered yoga after a long career as a Radiologist and medical author.

His continued desire to help people led him to the Kripalu yogic philosophy of self-observation without judgment and the practice of kindness and compassion. He writes from his personal experience of the transformative effects of yoga that helped him to overcome an inflexibility of body and mind in the pursuit of a meaningful yoga practice.

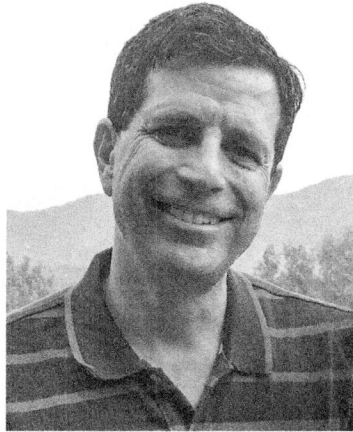

His first book, *Journey Into Yoga ~ A Guide for Transformation and Discovery,* is an exploration of yoga for beginning practitioners, those that have always wanted to do yoga, but haven't for any number of reasons, and anyone wanting to deepen their practice. The book presents the proper mindset to overcome the obstacles to a regular yoga practice, a comprehensive overview of the philosophy, human anatomy, and the science of yoga, as well as the *asanas* and *pranayama,* all to enhance one's experience.

He is a graduate of Hofstra University, New York University School of Medicine, and the Kripalu Center for Yoga and Health.

He and his wife, Lauren, split their time between the serenity of beautiful Cape Cod and the energy and excitement of Boston. His two sons, daughter, daughter-in-law, son-in-law and grandson all live in the Boston area.

You can learn more about Gordon at:

https://www.gkanzeryoga.com

ALSO BY GORDON KANZER, MD

Journey Into Yoga ~

A Guide for Transformation and Discovery